ASTHMA &
HAY FEVER

Dr Allan Knight is a medical consultant who specializes in allergies. He is head of the Division of Clinical Immunology at Sunnybrook Medical Centre in Toronto and a Professor at the University of Toronto.

He does research on new drugs for allergies and asthma along with carrying a major teaching and consulting load. He still finds time to play tennis regularly and to travel all over the world.

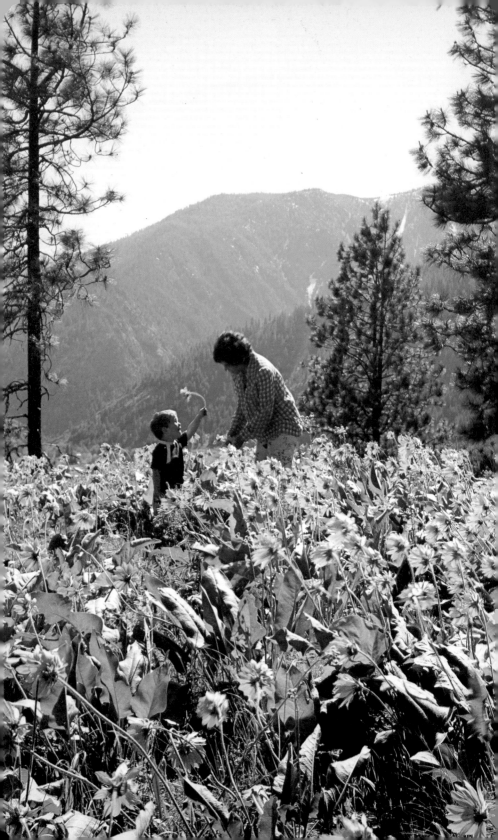

ASTHMA &
HAY FEVER
How to relieve
wheezing and sneezing

ALLAN KNIGHT
BSc, MD, CM, FRCP(C), FACP

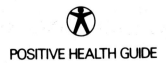

POSITIVE HEALTH GUIDE

© Dr Allan Knight 1981

First published in the United Kingdom in 1981
by Martin Dunitz Limited, London
This edition published in 1991 by
Macdonald Optima, a division of
Macdonald & Co. (Publishers) Ltd

A member of Maxwell Macmillan Pergamon Publishing Corporation plc

British Library Cataloguing in Publication Data
Knight, Allan
    Asthma and hay fever. — 2nd ed.
    1. Man. Hay fever. Self-treatment.   2. Man. Bronchi. Asthma. Self
    treatment
    I. Title   II. Series
    616.202068

    ISBN 0-356-19772-7

Macdonald & Co. (Publishers) Ltd
Orbit House
1 New Fetter Lane
London EC4A 1AR

Printed and bound in Singapore

CONTENTS

To my patients
who have taught me so much.

FOREWORD

Professor Jack Pepys
MD, FRCP, FRCPE, FRCPath, FACCP

Emeritus Professor of Clinical Immunology, University of London

Asthma is a common disorder and its diagnosis often causes much anxiety, for parents of asthmatic children in particular. It is as well to appreciate that it can vary widely in severity ranging from mild, occasional episodes of minor importance to severe incapacitating illness. It is often found in children, simply as a persistent, irritating cough more troublesome to the parents than the child. Perhaps, more than in most other illnesses, an understanding of how it comes about and how to manage it are of immediate importance to the patient in whose own hands much of its day-to-day control lies.

This comprehensive, commonsense and readily understandable account of the relevant aspects of asthma and hay fever is clearly provided here by Dr. Allan Knight. He is widely experienced in this field and is highly respected both nationally and internationally. He has performed a most useful service by providing patients and their families with a proper perspective for these two common conditions for their guidance. He is to be congratulated for supplying in this book the type of continuing, informed support which may not otherwise be readily available. I have no doubt that *Asthma and hayfever* will not only help thousands of patients but should also be of assistance to the doctors and nurses who treat them.

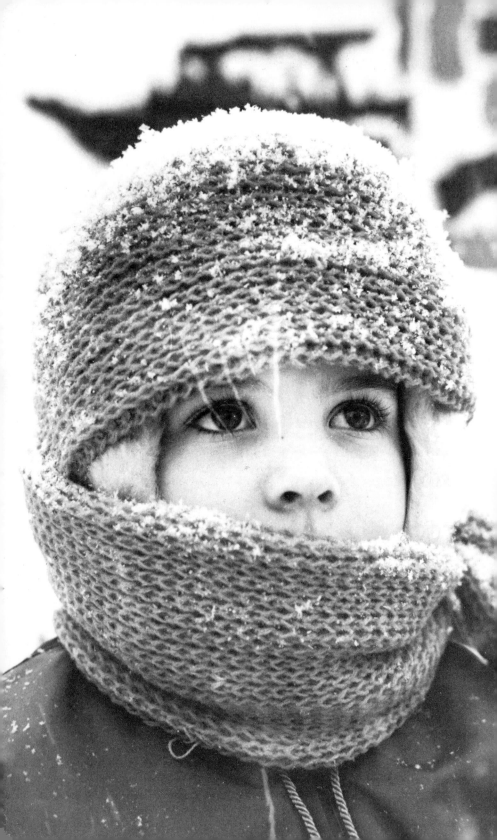

INTRODUCTION

Most of us take our bodily functions for granted. Things go along automatically and we don't have to think about them. We digest the food we eat without difficulty or deliberate effort. Our hearts beat regularly and keep us going. And all the time we breathe air in and out without even thinking about it. Until something goes wrong. Suddenly breathing isn't easy any more. And then we do start to think and to worry about it. Is it serious? Will we get worse? Might we even become invalids?

The answer is almost certainly no. It depends in part, of course, on what has gone wrong and how seriously. But there is also a lot we can do ourselves to overcome the causes of our shortness of breath and its effects on our general health.

There are many possible reasons why we might feel breathless. Our noses can plug up, or our breathing passages block, or our lungs become damaged in a variety of ways. This book is designed to explain just what is going wrong in the cases of asthma and hay fever.

Both conditions are very widespread. 10 to 20 per cent of the population of the Western world suffers from problems with the nose and 3 to 5 per cent from asthma or asthmatic bronchitis. If you are among these many sufferers you will almost certainly want to know something about what is making you sneeze or wheeze and what you can do to relieve it.

Can we do anything about it? Yes, indeed. Provided first of all we face the problem and find out what is bringing it on. In many cases we don't know exactly what causes it, but it could be, for example, an allergy, or the irritation caused by cigarette smoke or industrial pollution. A common cold, like many other infections, always makes things worse and may even be the cause of an attack of asthma or hay fever. Keeping generally fit, eating a good diet and taking enough exercise can all do a lot to make us less vulnerable to these infections. Also we must never forget the important part played by our emotions on our bodies. Good emotional health helps keep us physically fit. And vice versa.

The enormous amount of time lost from work or school as a result of asthma, hay fever and other nose or sinus problems makes it worth everyone's while to look for ways to avoid these illnesses. And the cost of hospital time and services used in the treatment of asthma and bronchitis make the roles of prevention and self-help especially important. This is not, of course, to say that you should not consult your doctor about the problem. He will be able to give you a great deal of help and you should certainly never embark on any treatment programme without first getting his advice.

I shall try in this book to explain first how we breathe normally and then what can go wrong and why. I hope also to show that there are many ways you can help reduce these problems, or even avoid them altogether. It is certainly worthwhile to try, and the benefits of success will be great.

1. HOW WE BREATHE

Breathing is necessary for life. All the cells in our bodies depend on oxygen in order to work normally. This oxygen, taken from the air around us, is delivered to the blood through our lungs. It passes through our mouths or noses down into the bronchial tree and then out through the walls of the lungs into the blood. The blood stream then carries the oxygen (attached to the red blood cells) to the different parts of our body where it is used to produce energy for all our activities. The waste products, mainly carbon dioxide, are then carried back to our lungs and exhaled when we breathe out.

What does the nose do?

Although the nose's function is not necessary for life, since we can also get air to our lungs through our mouths, we do breathe more easily, efficiently and comfortably if the air is allowed to pass first through our nostrils. The nose will, among other things, heat, humidify and filter all the air which is breathed in through it. When you consider the wide range of conditions, including extremes of heat and cold, areas of very high or very low humidity and often of dense pollution, in which your nose has to work, it is amazing that most people get along as well as they do without trouble.

The nose is also of course the area for our sense of smell. This is not nearly as acute or effective in humans as it is in animals. Nonetheless, the pleasures of being able to smell a bouquet of flowers or the aroma of a fine wine or of an exotic dish speak for themselves, and those unfortunate people among us who have lost their sense of smell miss these pleasures greatly. On the other hand, of course, they don't have to experience the many unpleasant smells that surround us.

Each nostril contains three finger-like pieces of bone surrounded by a very active lining where the work of the nose goes on. The lining is covered by a thin layer of mucus which acts as a protective coat to help in conditions of excessive dryness and which contains enough water to dampen the inhaled air if necessary. This mucus layer also helps protect the lining from viruses and bacteria which can cause infection.

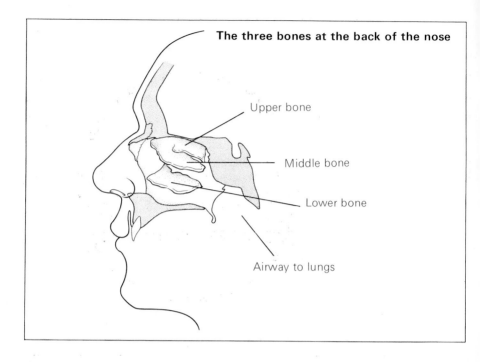

The three bones at the back of the nose

Upper bone

Middle bone

Lower bone

Airway to lungs

The lining has a cover of tiny hairs which waft the mucus outwards. These are necessary for cleansing the air before it gets to our lungs. Most importantly the normal nose lining acts as a filter, sponging up potentially harmful gases, chemicals or solid particles. If any of these reached the bronchial tubes they would cause a coughing spell as the lower airway then tried to get rid of them. If they reached even further, to the more sensitive area of the lungs, they might cause inflammation or possibly permanent damage.

Several things can interfere with the lining of the nose and stop it carrying out its useful protective role. The following are particularly common culprits which you should try to avoid:
- the very dry air created in overheated houses or factories;
- smoking (nicotine can actually poison the nasal tissues and the burning of both paper and tobacco acts as a strong irritant);
- over-use of certain nose drops or nose sprays;
- infections.

What are sinuses?

We cannot discuss the nose without also considering the sinuses, which can sometimes become infected and are often blamed for people's headaches. We have several sinuses, which are air-filled spaces designed to

The lining

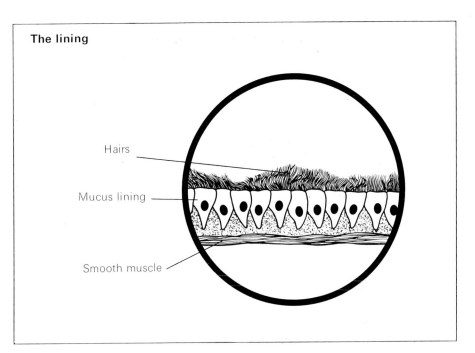

Hairs

Mucus lining

Smooth muscle

The sinuses

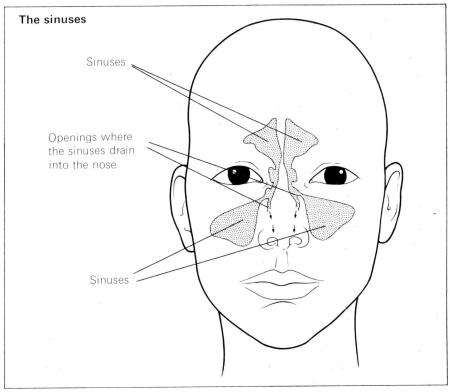

Sinuses

Openings where the sinuses drain into the nose

Sinuses

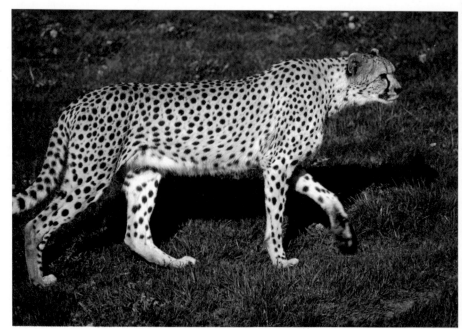

Sinuses are not essential to breathing. Four-legged animals do not have them at all.

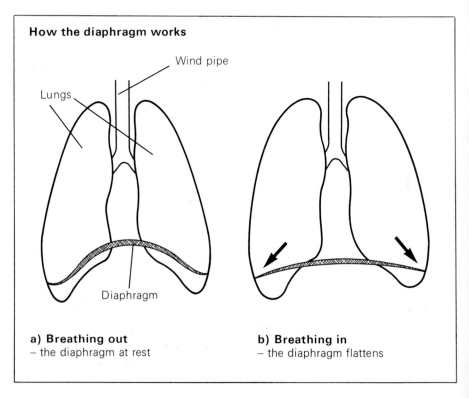

How the diaphragm works

Wind pipe

Lungs

Diaphragm

a) Breathing out
– the diaphragm at rest

b) Breathing in
– the diaphragm flattens

lighten the weight of our skulls. If our skulls were solid bone it would be very difficult for us to hold our heads up, particularly since we walk on two feet. Four-legged animals have a lower centre of gravity than we do which means that the weight of their skulls is less important and they don't need sinuses.

Just at the back of our noses are the paranasal sinuses. They have a lining identical to the lining in the nose I have just described, with just the same kind of cleansing mechanism. There is an opening from these sinuses to the nose for drainage, and it is when these openings become blocked, because of an allergy or an infection, that pressure builds up and may cause you pain.

How do our lungs work?

The act of respiration is a sort of bellows movement, with all the main effort being put into inhaling, followed by an automatic relaxing of the stretched lungs to their normal size when we breathe out. As the air is drawn in, the volume of our lungs increases, mainly by the action of the muscles of the diaphragm. Then the rib cage returns to its original size, and as it does so it pushes the air back out.

The anatomy of the lung is like that of a leafy tree, except it is upside down. The trunk of the tree corresponds to the largest airway which forms the wide tube in our necks coming down from our nose and mouth. This upper airway then divides into two tubes leading to the left and right lungs. These in turn subdivide many times like the branches of a tree, each subdivision getting narrower than the last. And indeed the tubes are known, appropriately enough, as the bronchial tree.

All the tubes are covered by a thin surface lining with the same kind of protective mucus blanket and tiny hairs as the lining in the nose. These two kinds of protection, along with our ability to cough, help keep the airways free of harmful particles.

How the bronchial muscles work

All the air tubes, both the large (bronchi) and the small (bronchioles), have walls made up of spiral bundles of so called smooth muscle. This is quite different from the striped muscles (such as those of the neck, limbs or back) which help us move or keep steady. We can control the action of striped muscle deliberately. For example, when we want to walk we do so by using the appropriate muscles in our legs. These muscles have a constant state of tension called tone, which enables us to maintain our normal posture and balance even during sleep (although all our muscles do relax to some degree at that time).

The lungs and the bronchial tree

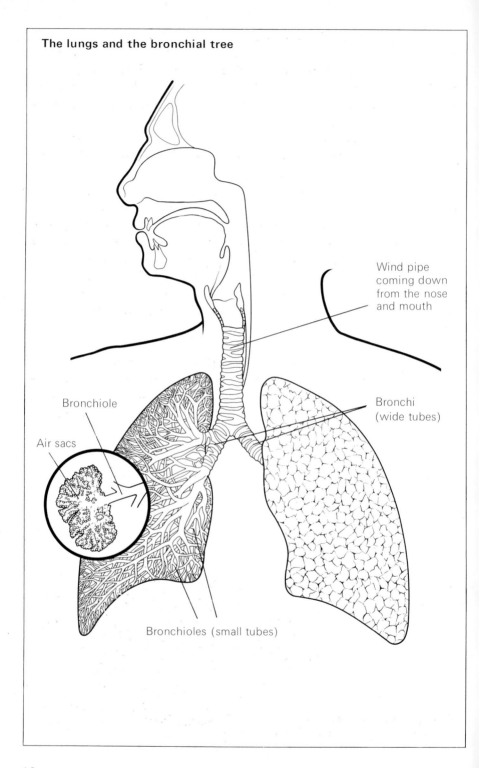

Wind pipe
coming down
from the nose
and mouth

Bronchiole

Air sacs

Bronchi
(wide tubes)

Bronchioles (small tubes)

Smooth muscle, on the other hand, is not under our voluntary control. It keeps working whether we think about it or not. It too has a tone or state of tension like a spring coil. This tone can be affected by emotional stress as we shall see later. Smooth muscle works with a type of sinuous movement which carries on all the time and pushes things automatically along the tube it surrounds.

This kind of muscle is, by the way, present in all our arteries as well as in a number of other parts of our bodies such as our intestines and the tubes which carry urine to our bladders.

The tone of the bronchial tree, like all smooth muscle, is regulated by a specialized part of the brain which controls all the things we do automatically – such as breathing, or pumping the blood around our bodies. In the bronchial tree messages going to and from this part of the brain influence the size of the tubes carrying the air. If one type of message is sent the tubes get wider and air moves more freely in and out of the lung. If the opposite influence takes over, the width reduces and it will be more difficult to breathe. This is particularly important in asthma as we shall see later.

How oxygen gets from the lungs to the blood stream

At the farthest ends of the bronchial tubes are many tiny air sacs. These correspond to the leaves in our tree analogy. The lining of each sac is very thin and close by is a tiny blood channel. It is here that the vital gas

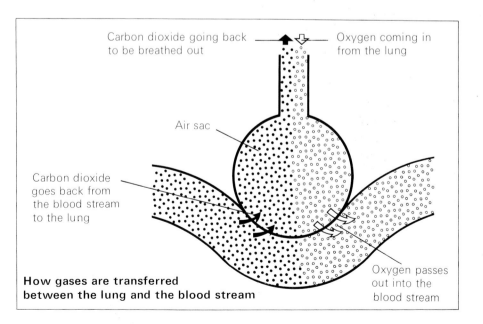

Carbon dioxide going back to be breathed out

Oxygen coming in from the lung

Air sac

Carbon dioxide goes back from the blood stream to the lung

Oxygen passes out into the blood stream

How gases are transferred between the lung and the blood stream

exchange takes place. Oxygen is transferred from the air sac to the blood through the thin membrane and is carried to all parts of the body where it helps produce energy. A major waste product is carbon dioxide. This gas travels back in the reverse direction to the oxygen, getting transferred from the blood to the air sac. It is then breathed out through the mouth and nose.

Normal breathing depends, then, not only on the nostrils and sinuses being in good order, but also on the normal working of these little air sacs.

Measuring breathing

When we come to look at the abnormal states of breathing caused by asthma and hay fever later in the book, it may be helpful to understand something of the ways in which we can measure breathing. This can often give a more precise clue to someone's breathing difficulties than can be gained from either his or his doctor's impression. Measuring levels of breathing may show that the problem is either more or indeed less serious than we thought. This can give us a better guide towards finding the right treatment.

The mechanics of breathing depend on many factors including a person's height, weight, age and sex. A tall person will have larger lung volumes than someone who is shorter, and a man generally has larger volumes than a woman. Children, having smaller bodies, naturally have smaller lungs than adults. And the elderly perform less well than younger people as their muscles get weaker and less elastic. All in all the person who should perform best is a young male athlete in the prime of training and who is not a smoker. But special exercise programmes can improve anybody's breathing to some degree.

The nostrils are much less important to your breathing than the lungs. It is possible to measure the flow of air through one or both nostrils, but this depends on so many things and can vary so much even from one minute to the next that we don't bother with it very often unless it is part of a research project.

The most useful and simplest measure of how freely air is moving in and out of your bronchial tubes is known as the peak flow. This is the amount of air you can breathe out by blowing as hard as you can after completely filling your lungs. Provided the effort you put into this is kept reasonably constant each time you take the measurement, it is a handy and reliable way to tell how blocked your airways are. You can test it from day to day and at different times during the course of a single day. A mini peak flow meter made of plastic such as the one shown here can give you a

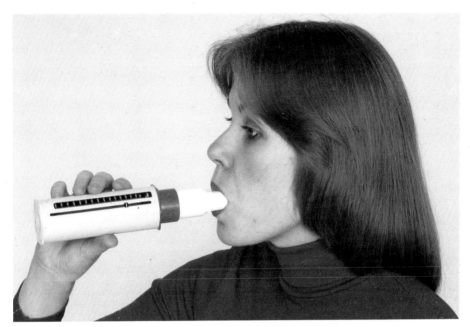

A peak flow meter which you can use to keep a regular check on your breathing.

reasonably accurate idea of how your asthma is progressing.

Many more measurements of the mechanics and other aspects of lung performance can be carried out but they are often complex and not readily available except at special centres so I shall not go into them here.

Changes in normal breathing patterns

While breathing is mostly automatic, we can of course make some voluntary adjustments to it, as for example when we breathe in to enjoy the smell of a lovely flower. When we pant with excitement or fear, it is sometimes intentional and sometimes not. Even fit people breathe more heavily after exercise. How out of breath we feel will depend on our state of health, how much we have smoked and how hard the exercise was.

High altitudes can also affect breathing. Things a mountain climber can do easily at moderate heights produce almost unbearable shortness of breath at very high altitudes where there is much less oxygen. Interestingly, people who live at high altitudes find that their bodies do adjust to this and they can breathe normally.

Occasionally anxious and frightened people hyperventilate – that is, they pant for no other reason than because they are feeling emotionally upset. If they continue doing this for several minutes they blow off

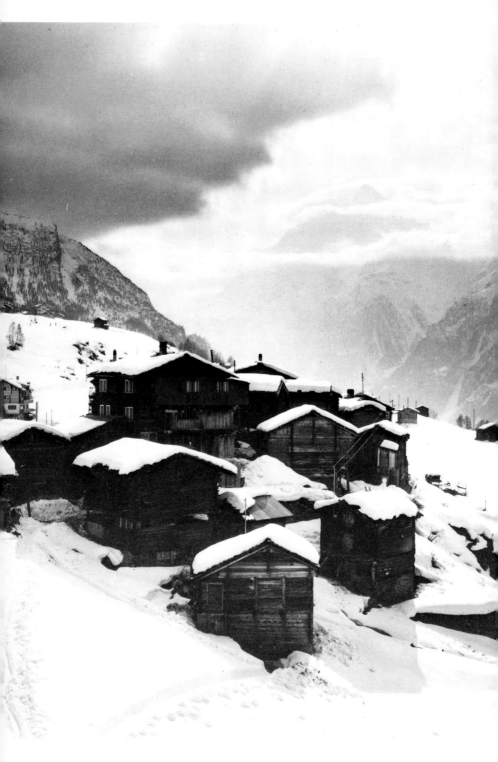

excessive amounts of carbon dioxide. This changes the amount of acid in their blood and they may feel quite dizzy or faint. As soon as they stop this so-called overbreathing the acid in the blood returns to normal levels and they feel better. Children sometimes learn to manipulate their parents by doing this. When they are overbreathing their carbon dioxide level tends to fall and the automatic drive to breathe may stop temporarily. If this happens the child turns blue. This is naturally very frightening, and the child may try to scare his parent deliberately to get his own way. Happily it does not last long and is no more serious than holding the breath – which is another method children may use to try getting their own way.

I hope this introductory explanation of the way we breathe will help you to understand better the problems we shall be looking at in the rest of the book. Some of these problems are of our own making and can be reversed. Others will respond to the right kind of treatment so that, even if we cannot cure them completely, we can at least learn the best way to bring them under control and manage to live with them.

People who live at high altitudes adjust to the reduced amount of oxygen in the air they breathe.

2. A WORD ABOUT ALLERGY

Not all symptoms of asthma or so-called hay fever are caused by allergy. But many are, and, before going on to talk about the specific problems, I think it would be a good idea to say something about just what we mean by allergy. It is a word that has been often misused and has led to considerable confusion.

What is an allergy?

The definition of allergy is 'altered reactivity to a specific substance', meaning that one person can react to something differently from his fellows and as a result become ill. The term should only be applied to someone who is sensitive to things which, for most people, do not produce any abnormal symptoms at all. It is really a hypersensitivity, since the poor person who is allergic becomes sick as a result of substances most people do not notice at all.

To use a specific example, we are all exposed from early life to the grass in meadows, lawns and parks. The various types of grasses pollinate at different times throughout the spring and summer and their pollen is breathed in by everyone around. Most people will not even be aware that it is in the air, but the 10 to 15 per cent of the population who are allergic to pollen will find, as soon as they inhale it, that they start getting the typical symptoms of sneezing, streaming eyes and so forth. They are the ones who have become sensitized.

What happens is this. The allergic person develops inside him a protein called an antibody, which is aimed at a specific irritant known as an allergen – in this case grass pollen. When this antibody comes in contact with the allergen they combine and various chemicals are released. The best known of these is histamine (hence the word anti-histamine for one of the drugs used in treatment). Wherever it is released, histamine will start an inflammation and cause swelling, redness and itching. If it is released in your nostrils, eyelids, or the lining of your bronchial tree this swelling and itching will cause sneezing, a runny nose, stuffiness, itchy eyes or coughing and wheezing – in other words an attack of hay fever or asthma.

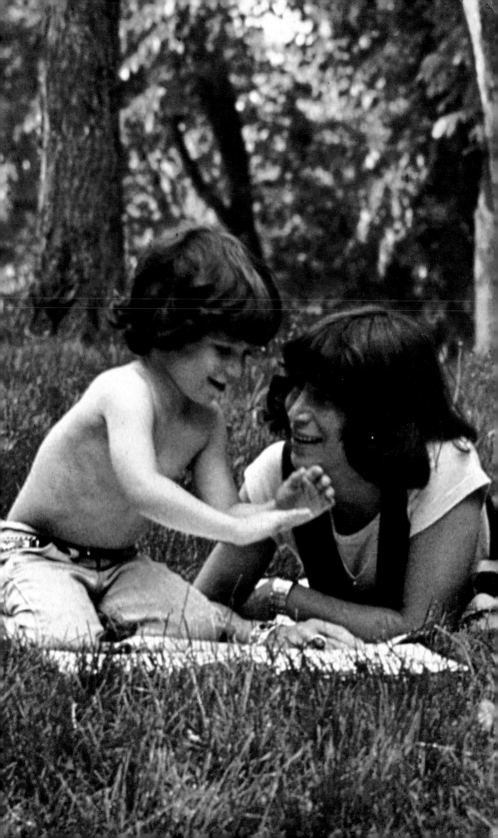

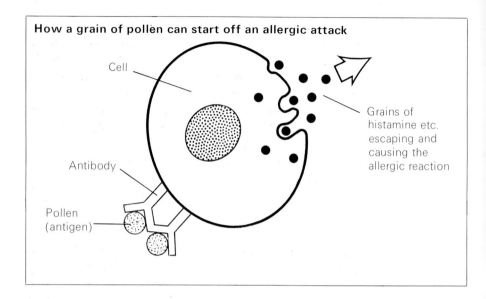

How a grain of pollen can start off an allergic attack

Cell

Grains of histamine etc. escaping and causing the allergic reaction

Antibody

Pollen (antigen)

Skin tests

We can find out whether or not you have got these antibodies by doing an allergy skin test. This means putting a small extract of the grass pollen, or whatever else is suspected of causing your reaction, onto your skin and then making a pinprick through it. If the person tested does have the specific antibody to that pollen, antibody and allergen will again combine, histamine will be released and it will create a small itchy swelling in the place where the prick was made. This will confirm that the person is allergic to that particular allergen.

These tests are not completely reliable and do not always match up with what the people being tested actually experience. Sometimes a person can get a positive result even though he does not suffer from hay fever or asthma. But in general the tests are quite a good guide to whether you have an allergy and, if so, what causes it.

Patterns of allergy

It has been known for many years that families who suffer allergic symptoms such as hay fever often follow a common pattern. They become allergic to a whole series of things in different ways from childhood on.

A typical case history is this. James at six months, shortly after getting a cold, shows his first sign of being prone to allergies. It begins as eczema – an inflammation of the skin which is itchy, red and moist, and occurs especially in the crease areas of the body such as the neck, elbows, groin and knees. After a time this eczema spontaneously disappears. (Changes in diet often receive undue credit for this 'cure'. It is true that cow's milk, eggs, wheat, and orange juice, among other foods, can make eczema worse but the disappearance of the problem may have nothing to do with food.) Once his eczema clears James then goes on to develop hay fever every summer, and this lasts till he is twenty-five. Occasionally, during a very bad season, he begins to wheeze.

Sometimes people seem to grow out of an allergy at puberty, but in many cases it will continue even into their thirties or later. Occasionally allergic children develop an asthmatic condition. This may similarly disappear at puberty, or in some cases it begins at this age, just as their hay fever clears up.

Many people are allergic to more than one thing and notice that their different allergies affect each other. When they have their hay fever, they may find they also become more sensitive to things which normally don't bother them. For instance they may get a very itchy mouth when they eat fresh melon during the pollen season, even though they can eat it without trouble during the winter months.

Why these patterns develop we are not sure, although it seems certain that the general tendency to develop allergies, whatever form they may take, is something that people inherit from their parents.

Common causes and what to do about them

Hay fever and asthma are most likely to be caused by the things we breathe in from the air around us. This can include many different substances, and knowing how best to tackle an allergy depends on discovering exactly what is causing it. The following are the allergens which most often give rise to problems.

Pollen

The commonest causes of hay fever are the pollens given off by certain plants during their particular pollinating season. These can also cause allergic asthma. Interestingly the pollens most likely to produce allergies come from what can only be described as ugly plants and weeds. Our beautiful flowers tend to have heavy pollen which does not spread far in the air and is carried for fertilization by bees or other insects. Ugly weeds on the other hand tend to have lighter pollen grains which are carried along the wind for long distances and can sensitize an allergic person even when he is far away from the original plant.

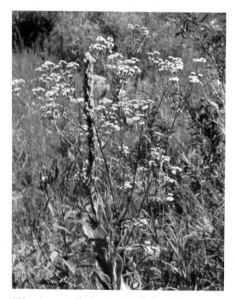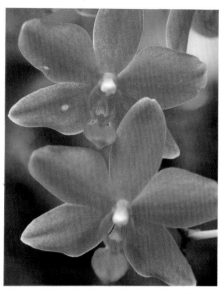

Weeds usually have small light pollen grains and are therefore more likely to bring on allergic attacks than are large showy flowers with heavy pollens.

The worst pollens for producing allergies are found in temperate climates. They include tree pollen, such as birch, which is a particular problem in Scandinavia and parts of Canada. Pine pollen can also have a very bad effect, but it is a heavy material and doesn't travel very far so you have to be quite close to the pine trees before getting the symptoms. Other notorious sensitizing pollens include all the many types of grasses, ragweed (which is a major allergy problem in most of North America but not in Europe) and mugwort, which is another common weed. In Britain and Europe grass pollen is the commonest cause of hay fever.

All of these pollens are only around during their own pollinating seasons, which are well recognized and depend to some extent on the geography and climate of the place where you live. By noticing exactly when your hay fever develops you can usually find out which pollen is causing it. If it is possible for you to avoid being in a particularly high pollen area at the critical time you may be able to avoid getting the symptoms. This of course is not always practicable, and if you cannot escape the pollen your best defence against it is likely to be the medicine described on pages 60 and 103.

Air-conditioning systems can be useful for filtering pollen out of the air – particularly in the bedroom.

Mould

Another one of the major factors in the air around us which can produce hay fever or asthma symptoms is something called mould. Moulds are members of the fungus family and are widely found in all non-polar countries. Not all of them cause allergy, but some do. They travel around in large numbers in the air, having spread from the soil – especially fields with crops. However as they are light and buoyant they can travel long distances away from their original source.

The existence of moulds and fungi has been known for half a century. Their potential for causing allergy has been recognized just as long. They are mainly found during the warmer months, but during the freezing weather they are still around – just lying dormant. As soon as the thaws begin in the spring they reappear and may last well into autumn. Even during the winter they may cause allergy symptoms indoors in the warm. Especially high levels of mould occur when there is rain or fog and in the damper conditions of nightfall. Because the moulds are most prevalent in the spring, summer and autumn people who are allergic to them are often mistakenly thought to be reacting to the pollen around at the same time of the year.

It is only the smaller sized fungi which cause allergy. The bigger particles get trapped by the defences in our noses and bronchial trees and

Newly ploughed fields are warm and damp – an ideal environment for allergy-inducing moulds.

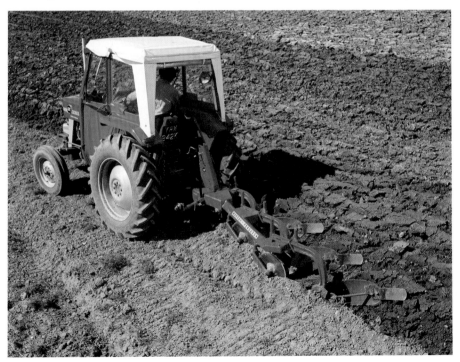

we cough or sneeze to get rid of them. The smaller ones can get through these protective barriers and so reach the sensitive linings where they set up an allergic reaction, and cause the streaming itchy nose and eyes or the onset of an attack of wheezing, which all sufferers know so well.

The moulds flourish in warm, damp places and so are especially common in soil, trees, plants, still water, animal hair and damp basements. They can even invade and grow in air conditioning ducts, poorly maintained cold air vaporizers or humidifiers, and this is a source which is easily missed. They occur in higher density in forests than in open countryside, and well kept lawns are also a favourite habitat. When the lawn is cut or raked over to gather leaves these moulds can be spread very far afield. Lawn mowing is a chore the allergic person has a good excuse to avoid! Similar hazards face him if he has to work with silage or compost heaps or leaf and peat mulches.

Indoors, moulds are found not only in musty basements, as I mentioned earlier, but also in food storage areas, soiled upholstery and garbage containers. They are also found in cotton, kapok and wallpaper. They love to grow in old foam rubber which tends to retain moisture. Synthetic foams, if moist, will also become contaminated after a time. It is very difficult to get rid of the moulds, so any objects you suspect of harbouring them will have to be removed from the home, school or work place as this is the only way to prevent allergic problems arising from these little fungi.

House dust

This is such a normal part of all our lives and is so often blamed for various allergies that it is worth a special discussion. Remember that house dust consists of many different substances, so it is very difficult to think of it as just one specific allergen. It is made up of a mixture of coarse and fine particles. The coarse bits will cause anybody, allergic or not, to cough and sneeze – just as breathing in ground pepper will do. Almost anyone will find his nose, eyes and throat irritated when cleaning out a dusty attic, but the symptoms are usually mild and brief. Only if you have the twitchy lungs of asthma are you likely to start coughing and wheezing very badly when you inhale a lot of dust.

Allergic symptoms, however, are something different. As in the case of moulds they are always produced by the smaller particles, invisible to the naked eye. These are the only ones that can get through all your breathing defences and, if you are allergic to them, make the linings of your nose or lungs swell and itch.

What is in dust? There may be pollens from grass, trees or weeds which have been transferred to the house. The skin scales, dander, hair, or even

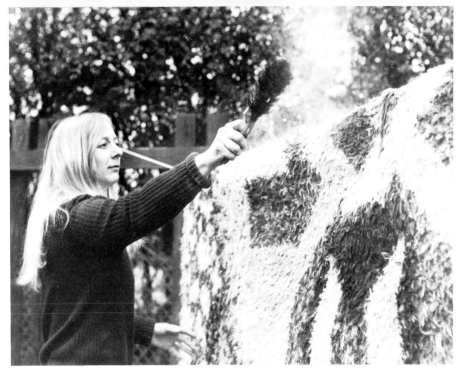

If you are allergic to dust you would do well to stay out of the way when any spring cleaning is being done.

the dried saliva from the family pet certainly gets into the household's dust, as do fragments shed from various kinds of clothing. There may also be tiny bits of paper from the newspaper and there will almost certainly be shreds from cigarette paper and tobacco if anyone has been smoking.

Dust may also contain dead insects, bacteria from the skin, fibres from plant or animal matter, food remnants from last month's supper, debris from old upholstered furniture, dry wood particles from chairs or firewood, soot from the neighbour's chimney and ash from the fireplace. Obviously dust contains such a myriad of potential allergens that it is a difficult trick to pinpoint which ones among them may be causing somebody's allergic reactions.

The best way to manage if you have an allergy to dust is of course to keep your environment as dust-free as possible, particularly in the bedroom. But keeping a house free from dust is easier said than done. Try to avoid having thick pile carpets, upholstered furniture, or folded drapes, all of which can hold dust. Old books, libraries and poorly ventilated rooms are all great dust traps too.

The bedroom of an allergic person, particularly a child, should have a plain hardwood floor which should be vacuumed regularly and mopped with a damp mop. It is best to have non-upholstered furniture, a reasonably new synthetic foam mattress, perhaps in a washable plastic

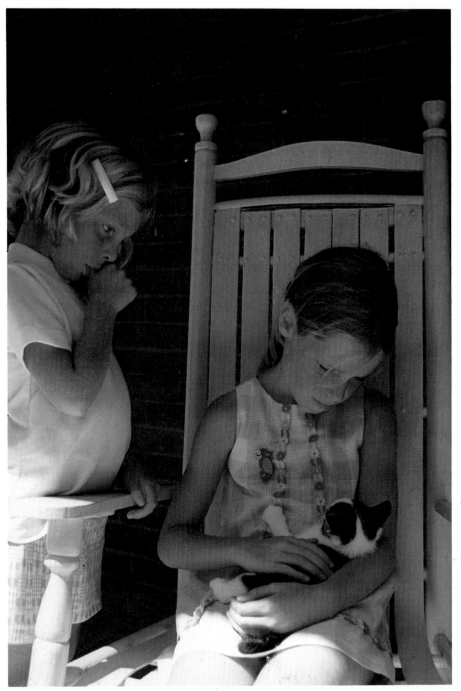

Animal fur is a common cause of allergy. If you suffer from asthma or hay fever all the year round it may be being brought on by your family pet.

cover, and to avoid feathers in pillows and quilts as these also tend to contain a lot of dust. Old stuffed toys should be removed from the bedroom as they become mouldy and usually dusty as well with age. Above all the bedroom should be well ventilated and free from any unnecessary clutter. Any measures you can take along these lines should do a lot to reduce allergic attacks due to dust.

Mites: Interestingly studies done during the last decade, at first in Holland and then in Britain and Japan, have shown that, in these countries at least, the main cause of house dust allergy is a microscopic insect called a mite. Mites live on human skin and are shed with the old skin scales onto bedding and clothing. This has not been as great a problem in North America or alpine areas of Europe, where the climate and housing arrangements are different. Holland, Britain and Japan are low lying land masses at sea level with weather that is humid and neither very hot nor very cold. In addition the houses in these countries are older than those in, say, North America or Australia, and central air conditioning is not as common. As mites flourish in damp, temperate places they are less prevalent in rooms kept dry by central heating systems or in countries where the climate is hot and dry.

As you cannot alter the climate of the place where you live the best way to reduce the mite problem is to bend every effort to keep the dust content down in your home and to make sure the house is as well heated and ventilated as possible.

Pets

Another common cause of allergic symptoms such as asthma or hay fever is the fur, or sometimes the skin scales or saliva, of a pet dog or cat. The fur from other animals such as guinea pigs, hamsters, horses and so on can also produce allergic reactions, as can bird feathers.

As long as the pet is around the symptoms will go on. No matter how well you dust and clean and vacuum or use air conditioners or other filtering systems you cannot get rid of the particles from the pet's coat which are making you sneeze or wheeze. The only thing you can do is to give the pet away. This can be a heart-rending thing to do, especially in the case of a child who is allergic to a pet which he dearly loves, but unfortunately there is really no other way to make the allergic symptoms subside.

If you are not sure that it is the pet that is causing the problems you can try giving it to someone else to look after for a few months to see whether this cures the allergy. Then, if it turns out not to be due to the animal, you will not have to cause the distress of getting rid of it unnecessarily.

Food

Food allergy does not often seem to produce hay fever symptoms. Many people sneeze after eating a very large meal or when drinking a bowl of hot soup or a glass of alcohol, but these sneezing spells are not caused by an allergy. They seem to be more a reflex action from the overfilled stomach or from the nose which has been warmed up by the hot soup or the alcohol. This reflex sneezing is apparently triggered off by a nerve pathway in the nose. (Many non-allergic people get reflex sneezing, as for example, when they first step outdoors into bright sunlight.)

Asthma can sometimes be caused by certain foods. Some people react with coughing, wheezing or sneezing after eating such things as wheat, milk or eggs or some of the dyes and preservatives added to manufactured foods. Nuts, eggwhite and shellfish are other common triggers. The major danger with this kind of allergic reaction is that the airway will become blocked, which is a serious problem and needs to be promptly treated with adrenalin.

The symptoms of food allergy will often include swollen lips and tongue and perhaps also a rash or an upset stomach as well as wheezing or coughing. It is much more common among children than adults, but even then is fairly rare.

The only thing you can do about food allergies is to avoid eating whatever affects you. The offending foods causing asthma are usually easily identified. For example, every time the child drinks milk, or eats chocolate or corn or fresh fruit or whatever it is, he is likely to start wheezing within a few minutes afterwards. Allergy skin tests for food are not reliable, so it is up to the alert parent to notice what is causing the problem and then cut that particular food out of the child's diet. In most cases the child will grow out of the allergy after a few years.

Allergy shots or injections

The purpose of these injections is to make you less sensitive to whatever is causing your hay fever or asthma and so reduce the symptoms. They are more commonly used in North America than in Britain or Australia. They are very tiny doses of a fairly diluted extract of the pollen or other allergen. The dose is gradually increased as you build up a resistance to it. The reason for starting with a low dose is safety. These are powerful substances which, if given in too large quantities, could be harmful.

Generally speaking allergy shots work best for children and young adults. Asthmatics after the age of forty rarely get any benefit from them. They work best if they are aimed at a pollen allergy, such as one to trees or grasses or weeds. They are sometimes effective in treating allergy to house

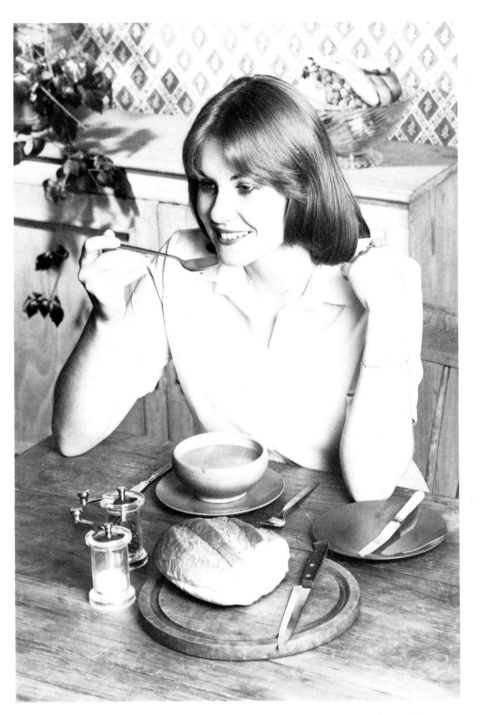

Hot soup can sometimes make you sneeze, but this is usually just a reflex action.

dust, particularly if the mite is the major factor. They can help with allergy to mould or household pets, although in the second instance it is better to remove the pet from your environment. They work best for hay fever. Results with asthma are often disappointing.

I cannot emphasize too strongly that for allergy shots to work at all, they must be specific. That is, if you have an allergy to grass pollen, only grass shots will work well. It is therefore most important that the doctor gets the diagnosis right. Sometimes, however, it is not easy to be precise. For instance, as I have pointed out, dust contains too many factors to make it possible to analyze a dust allergy exactly unless it is caused by mites. I feel that too many patients get allergy shots which don't do any good simply because the cause of their symptoms has not been properly identified.

The shots should be given for three to five years and then stopped while your condition is reassessed. Usually they are given once a week for about six months as the dose is very cautiously increased. After that they may be given every two weeks for several months and then the frequency cut to what is called a 'maintenance programme' of one injection a month.

Some patients notice that they get mild or even moderate attacks of asthma after an allergy shot. This is dangerous. If it happens to you the dose should be drastically cut or, if necessary, stopped altogether.

As an aside I always urge my patients to inquire as to what exactly is being used in the shots. You owe it to yourself to know what you are getting.

3. ASTHMA-THE FACTS

Roughly three out of every hundred people in the Western world suffer from asthma. In other places, such as Africa and among Canadian Indians it seems to be quite rare. But sometimes the figures are unreliable and in places where asthma has been considered rare this has later turned out to be simply because no one had carried out any proper studies. Recently, for example, a group went out from Australia to Papua New Guinea, where there was not supposed to be much asthma, and found by accurate breathing measurements that it was in fact quite a common problem.

Asthma causes a huge loss in working days, as studies in both Britain and North America have noted, so it has a considerable economic as well as a personal importance.

It is slightly more frequent in cities than in rural areas, and affects people of all ages. It is a particularly major problem among children. In about 30 per cent of cases it starts before the age of ten. It rarely starts after sixty. It may be quite a benign condition and many a patient wheezes happily into old age without undue discomfort.

Among children under the age of ten, asthma affects twice as many boys as girls. In the intermediate age group it affects men and women almost equally and in the older population it tends to show a slightly greater incidence among women.

What happens during an attack

Defining exactly what asthma is is difficult because its symptoms and causes can vary so much. Basically it is characterized by repeated sudden attacks of shortness of breath and audible wheezing – especially when you breathe out. Your chest feels tight and often you get a cough which is either dry or produces very little phlegm (unless there is added infection). What phlegm there is is clear – usually white or colourless. The most important point about asthma is that it is a temporary, reversible condition. Once the attack is over your bronchial tubes return to normal and you should be able to manage perfectly well once again.

It happens because of three things going on in your lungs at the same time, all of which combine to make the opening in the bronchial tubes get narrower, and so make it more difficult for the air to flow in and out:

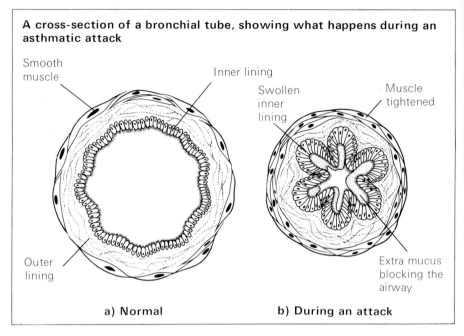

A cross-section of a bronchial tube, showing what happens during an asthmatic attack

Smooth muscle

Inner lining

Swollen inner lining

Muscle tightened

Outer lining

Extra mucus blocking the airway

a) Normal   b) During an attack

1. The smooth muscles of the bronchial tree get tight.
2. The glands under the lining of the air tubes give out more mucus than usual.
3. The inside wall of the tubes swells up.

If treated quickly all these things can be put back to normal by means of medication and the breathing exercises which I shall describe in the next chapter.

What you must not do is to allow the attack to continue unattended while it gets gradually worse and worse. If a serious attack goes on too long all your breathing muscles will have to work very hard and so become tired. In addition not enough oxygen will be getting to your blood stream and this will be another major cause of fatigue. The mucus in the bronchial tubes will become dry and hard because you will usually be breathing hard through your mouth and have neither the time or the appetite to drink enough liquids.

It takes time, indeed several days, to reach this stage, but if you ever did let an attack develop until it became this serious it could mean that you would need a mechanical ventilator or breathing machine to help get air into your lungs.

The answer is that it should never be allowed to happen. The golden rule is to start treating an attack of asthma as quickly as possible after it begins, and call a doctor if the regular treatment has no effect and you start getting worse instead of better.

Why are some people asthmatic and others not?

In the past asthma was often, quite unfairly, believed to be a self-induced problem, or a psychosomatic one. Certainly emotional factors can have an important effect, and I shall go on to discuss these later. Also many adults who had asthma in childhood confide later that they could bring on an attack, especially when they wanted to get round their parents, or avoid going to school or doing sports. However, while both these points are undoubtedly true, it should be said that nobody can have an attack of wheezing unless they do already suffer from a basic asthmatic problem.

This proneness to asthma stems from a (usually inherited) state of 'twitchy' lungs. The twitch is not actually in the lung tissues themselves but in the bronchial tubes. In the case of asthmatics the smooth muscle around the tubes is abnormally sensitive and will react by becoming tight or going into spasms whenever it is irritated by such things as allergies, chest infections, emotional stress, noxious fumes (especially cigarette smoke), exercise, coughing or even laughing hard.

In the case of the asthmatic person there are several different factors which contribute to these 'twitchy lungs' or bronchial hyperresponsiveness. Signals sent by the trigger factors mentioned earlier act on a variety of tissue cells in the area and on nerve endings which in turn release many more chemicals than we were aware of years ago. These chemicals all contribute to the swelling of the tubes and the increased mucus which is often produced by an attack of asthma. They also cause the muscles around the tubes to tighten further. The result is an inflamed, irritated swollen tissue which causes the asthma symptoms we recognise.

In the case of an asthmatic person two things seem to go wrong in these messages sent to the lungs. One is that the chemical which normally helps to keep the air tubes open gets partially blocked, so that it is less effective than usual. The other, which I think is even more important, is that too much of the opposite chemical is released, and this one contracts the airway and makes it narrower.

It seems that many asthmatic people are in a constant state of having tense muscles around their bronchial tubes, even when they feel quite well. This can be measured by some of the breathing tests I talked about in chapter one. Of course, there is a very wide range in the severity of asthma suffered by different people. Once they develop it some people have a constant wheeze. Others have perfectly normal breathing tests for most of the time, and only when they exercise vigorously, say by sprinting or

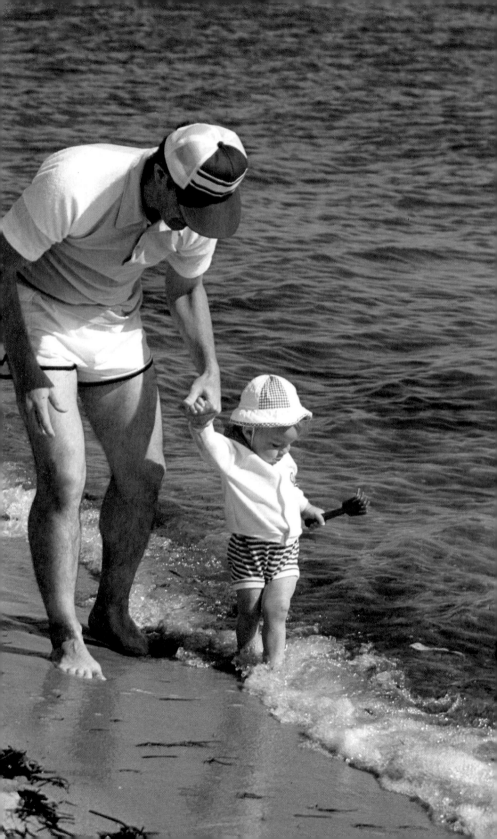

bicycling some distance into the wind, does an attack begin, usually subsiding again as soon as the exercise ends. Various types of food, especially dairy products, may also trigger asthma (see pages 50–53).

There are two main types of asthma. One is the kind which is triggered off by hypersensitivity to some specific factor such as pollen or animal fur. This is allergic asthma. The other, which is not allergic, does not have any such easily recognizable trigger. The two kinds have many different characteristics, and I shall discuss them separately.

Allergic asthma

There is usually a clear pattern to allergic asthma. It rarely starts after the age of forty, and almost always develops in childhood. In a typical case the child may well start off before he is a year old by developing eczema. Often during his first few years he will wheeze whenever he gets a cold. He also tends to be prone to croup – a chest infection which produces a deep, hacking, wheezing cough and some breathing difficulties. He may then seem to outgrow these, but goes on to develop perhaps some form of hay fever or an allergy to the family pet. When grass pollen is around in the summer he may find not only that he gets hay fever, with sneezing and a runny nose and itchy eyes, but also that he starts to wheeze and cough and feel tight in his chest. This is asthma.

The details I have already given in the last chapter about allergies and their causes all apply to this kind of asthma. It tends, by definition, to be seasonal and the person suffering from it only starts to wheeze at the times of year when the thing to which he is allergic is around. Sometimes of course people are allergic to things which are constantly around them, such as their pet cat or household dust or some substance produced at the place where they work. In these cases the allergic asthmatic attacks will continue throughout the year.

Allergic asthma is usually quite mild and responds easily to medical treatment or extra sleep or a few days away from whatever it is that is causing the problem. Trying to control dust, stopping smoking, giving away the pet to friends or perhaps moving away to a lakeside place for a week or two are all possible ways of helping. Allergy shots can also be effective in a few cases (see page 34).

Will you grow out of it?
There is a common feeling that children grow out of their asthma. This is true in about 50 per cent of cases. Of the others about half find that their

You may be able to get a respite from the worst of the pollen season by going to a lake or a seaside place.

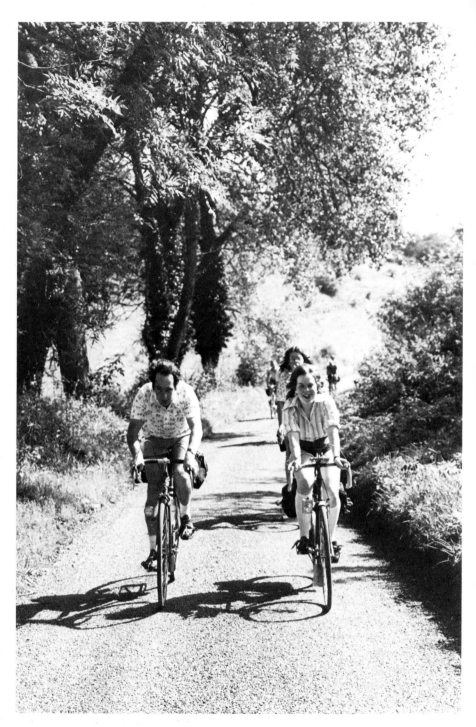

Vigorous cycling, particularly into a cold wind, can bring on non-allergic asthma.

asthma improves as they grow older, so that they only get occasional attacks, usually when they exercise or catch a bad cold. So only about one person in four with allergic asthma finds that he continues to wheeze into adulthood and has to go on taking regular treatment.

Non-allergic asthma

Unlike allergic asthma, which is commonest among children, the non-allergic kind most often begins after the age of forty.

A common case history would be that of an allergic child with hay fever and mild asthma who seems to grow out of his allergy at puberty. Everyone is pleased. But if we follow his life story further we often find that, at the age of about forty, he gets a heavy cold, begins to cough, and one night, out of the blue, he suddenly chokes up, and feels short of breath. He starts to wheeze and his asthma is back.

Non-allergic asthma does not only affect people who had asthma as children. It can come on quite suddenly in middle age, for example after you have been running for a bus in the cold or going out on a damp foggy night, or after you have had some sort of emotional shock. It commonly affects people who suffered a lot from bronchitis when they were young.

When the attack begins your chest feels constricted as though by a vice. The wheeze becomes quite noisy and some people feel as though they are having a heart attack. They may get over this first bout of wheezing fairly quickly, either by sitting down and resting until it wears off or by taking medicines. But the attacks do usually recur. Perhaps you will only get them on cold, humid or foggy nights, or when you exercise or catch a cold. The problem may not be incapacitating, but in some cases it may be. It need not mean that you have to start taking regular medicine, but in some cases it may. Non-allergic asthma seems to affect each person in a different way. There does seem to be some evidence to suggest there is a hereditary element in the condition, but it is nothing like as strong as in the case of allergic asthma.

A tense person is more likely to develop attacks than someone with a relaxed temperament. People who smoke and have chronic bronchitis are certainly likely to find that their asthma is worse.

Asthma at night

Asthma often seems to get worse at night and in the early morning. We don't know why this is but you may feel more comfortable and sleep better if you lie on two, or even three pillows rather than one. You may have more trouble breathing if you go to bed right after eating, and so common sense usually tells you not to take a meal at bedtime if you are prone to asthma.

If your bedroom is too hot or too dry this may make you cough, and so lead to an attack. You should do your best to make sure the room is well ventilated and kept at a comfortable temperature – neither too hot nor too cold.

Dangers in the air

Many things we breathe in can irritate the sensitive lining of our nose or chests even without causing an allergy. For example the chemical given out by your pet's fur could act directly on your bronchial tubes and set off an attack of asthma. So even if your condition is not allergic you would be well advised to keep your pet out of the bedroom. It could also be worth your while to keep dust down to a minimum, as the particles could irritate your lungs. Get rid of any feather pillows and perhaps also that hand-made feather or cotton quilt your grandmother gave you. However nice it may look it is probably giving off a lot of dust. All these things can also act as irritants and are substances you would do well to avoid whenever possible if you find that they bother you:

–frying foods
–fresh paint
–perfumes
–the smoke from a fire.

Cigarette smoke is of course another well known hazard. If you want a good night's sleep you would do well not to let your partner smoke, particularly in the bedroom.

Another major cause of asthmatic attacks, allergic and otherwise, is air pollution. The farmer may get asthma from his crops and soil dust or hay, or from the farm animals. Some of these he can avoid and others he can perhaps deal with by wearing a filtering mask over his nose and mouth. But the city dweller has to face the constant problem of diesel fumes from buses or trucks and the exhaust from automobiles and the belching smoke from factories, all filling the atmosphere with such irritants as carbon monoxide, sulphur dioxide and nitrous oxide. Ozone produced in the atmosphere is another irritating pollutant which can cause asthma. It is often produced by electronic filters which is why I do not recommend that people with asthma instal these gadgets in their homes.

The problems of infections

One of the commonest triggers for an attack of asthma in adults and children is a virus infection, which usually starts as a head cold. Feverish, flu-like illnesses which do not include the symptoms of a head cold do not

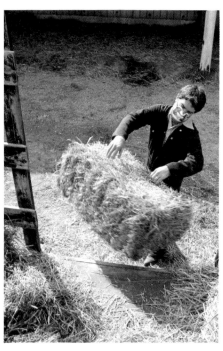
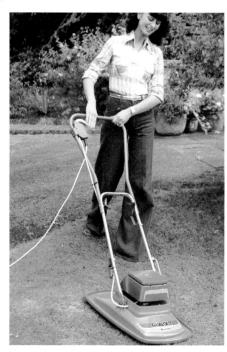

A farmer can wear a simple face mask to protect him from the dust in bales of hay.
Try to avoid grass cuttings, smoke or wet paint if any of them make you worse.

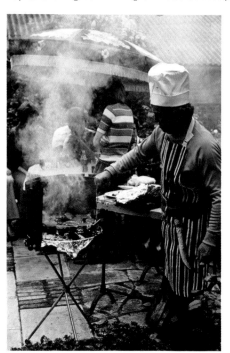
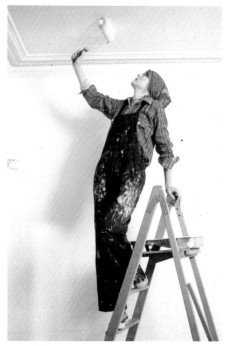

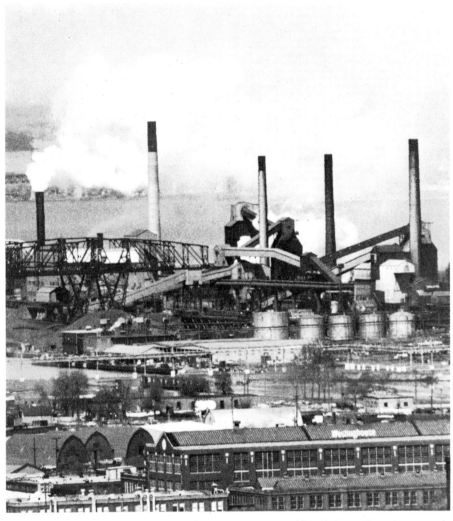

Industrial pollution can cause great irritation to the sensitive linings of our lungs and noses.

usually bring on asthmatic attacks. This suggests that what is important here is the inflammation in the nose, sinuses or bronchial tree which can cause a spasm in the lungs. Sometimes a viral cold goes on to become bronchitis which also causes wheezing.

Many patients with non-allergic asthma also have nasal polyps (see page 99). The reason these can cause asthma is that when they grow they block off the openings between the nose and the sinuses. This stops the sinuses from draining properly and so makes you more vulnerable to infection there. And, once again, infections in any part of the breathing passages can set off an attack of wheezing.

When drugs and chemicals make you wheeze
There is a well known set of symptoms which may arise when someone with nasal polyps and asthma takes an aspirin for a headache. He suddenly develops a very severe asthmatic attack and this becomes the pattern every time he takes an aspirin or other common pain relievers. It is not because he is allergic to aspirin but because it produces changes in the blood which affect the bronchial muscles and narrow his airways. The result is wheezing and shortness of breath.

The same kind of reaction has recently been shown to occur with other medicines. Some of the newer drugs used for arthritis may cause the same kind of attack in people predisposed to this kind of asthma. Also a family of chemicals called tartrazines which are often used as artificial colourings in food may do the same thing and should be avoided. (Tartrazines also occur naturally in some foods, mainly fresh fruit, but in such low concentrations that these foods rarely cause asthma.)

Curiously I have had the occasional patient who has told me that aspirin actually helps his asthma. This is not his imagination. His particular make-up is such that the action of aspirin happens to open up his bronchial tree rather than closing it down. He is fortunate indeed.

Asthma after a meal
Some people with asthma notice that they have an attack after a very large meal. This is probably because the overfilled stomach pushes up against the diaphragm and so there is less space in the chest for air. The attacks may also be due in part to acid regurgitation. If stomach acid leaks back into the throat, because of increased pressure in the stomach, it can make you cough, which may start an attack of asthma.

It is important, therefore, for anyone with asthma not to eat a lot at any one time and to avoid taking a meal just before sleeping. Getting an attack of asthma just when you go to bed is a particular nuisance, as it may interfere with your chances of a good night's sleep.

Is your job giving you asthma?

A newly discovered and major problem is that asthma can be directly related to all sorts of factors produced in our work environments. In our modern industrial society it is easy to see just how important and common the problem of dusts, gases and fumes, which can be carried long distances on the wind, could be. At least one highly reactive chemical known as

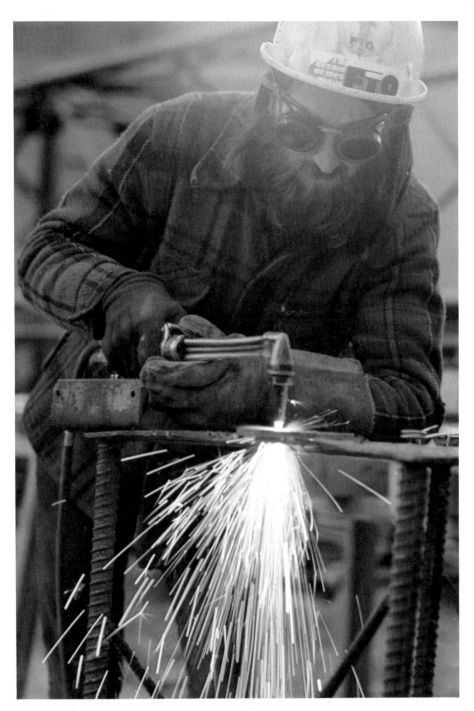

People sometimes get attacks of asthma as a result of doing a job which produces fumes or other irritating particles.

TDI which was previously only ever found in factories is now frequently used in the home in things like paints and plastics and also in do-it-yourself polyurethane foams. TDI has been blamed as a frequent cause of asthma. Industrial materials found at work can also be brought home in your clothing or hair or on your skin.

Grain handlers often get asthma from the dust on the farm or the freight cars transporting it. Metal workers may start to wheeze from the irritating oil of castor beans; photographic workers from platinum salts; bakers from flour dust, and so on. An interesting point is that the asthma may come on in the evening or during the night, several hours after the day shift is over. The reasons are only partly understood but delayed asthma is a common event and may make it harder for you to identify what has triggered it off.

Workers with occupational asthma often feel quite well on weekends and holidays, and only get their asthma again when they return to work. Such a pattern is an important clue to the real cause. So, if you have asthma, look at your job and see if there is anything there which may be contributing to it (other than your quick-tempered boss or the cigarette smoking colleague at the next desk).

Is exercise good for you?

In general the answer to this is yes. Unfortunately people do find that exercising makes their asthma worse. For instance granny may always start wheezing when she goes upstairs, even if she takes it slowly. Or an overweight person may well start wheezing with even modest exercise. But it is not only the elderly or the overweight who find this. People of any age, including children, can also tend to get wheezy when they exercise. The normal time lapse between taking the exercise and starting to wheeze is six minutes, but in some cases people find that they will start to wheeze several hours after finishing some strenuous exercise. However I feel that no asthmatic, whether or not physical effort makes him wheeze, should be put off taking exercise as, in the long run, it is sure to improve his breathing.

The amount of exercise you take may well have to be limited according to how bad your asthma is and what affects it. Some people feel worse on cold or damp days and so should try exercising indoors, or frequently but for short periods at a time. Some people find that they wheeze if they have to go uphill but are quite alright walking on the flat. Skiers may discover that it is only cross-country skiing that makes them wheeze and that they can go downhill with much less trouble. Whatever exercise you do you should take a dose of your regular medicine (either Intal or your bronchodilator) immediately before you begin. This will often prevent the asthma altogether.

There is an interesting aside to the subject of exercise-induced asthma. Many asthmatic athletes perform well even under the strenuous circumstances of competition, and only start to wheeze once the event is over. Just why this is so is not clear, but it appears that it may be related to the difference in temperature between their lungs and the outside air.

Most asthmatics, even bad ones, find that they can swim without getting an attack – particularly if they use a heated pool. We don't really know why this is but part of the reason may be that the buoyancy of the water is helpful to them and the warm moist air makes it easier to breathe.

A planned exercise programme should be approached reasonably and carefully. Casual, comfortable clothes make it easier to breathe than tight or confining ones. Some warming up before the exercise is a good idea and walking, running or jogging should be undertaken slowly at first and gradually increased with time over the days and weeks.

The rewards of feeling happier, healthier, more relaxed and more self-confident are well worth the effort and planning required. Most fit patients need fewer medicines than those who are unfit and they are less likely to be overweight.

Asthma and your diet

General fitness is also very important in keeping asthma under control, and this of course does depend on a healthy diet.

One important point is that people with asthma do well to keep slim. The depth of breathing in a fat person is usually shallow and he will become short of breath during even the mildest forms of exercise. Once an overweight person develops an attack of asthma it can be more serious and more difficult to overcome than in the case of a thin person, because of the extra work needed for obese people to move the air in and out of their lungs. Being overweight also puts an added burden on your breathing because extra oxygen will have to be carried to all the unnecessary fat cells.

Weight reduction is not always that simple. Medical knowledge about what causes obesity is still scant but there is no doubt that reducing the number of calories you take in will make you lose weight. The results are well worth the effort, but the overweight person will need constant encouragement to keep up the difficult and frustrating diet as well as any exercise programmes he may be doing alongside. It is almost sure to be a lifelong routine and should be planned that way.

On the other hand all of us need a certain minimum of nutrients. Eating too little can produce a state of relative starvation which may interfere

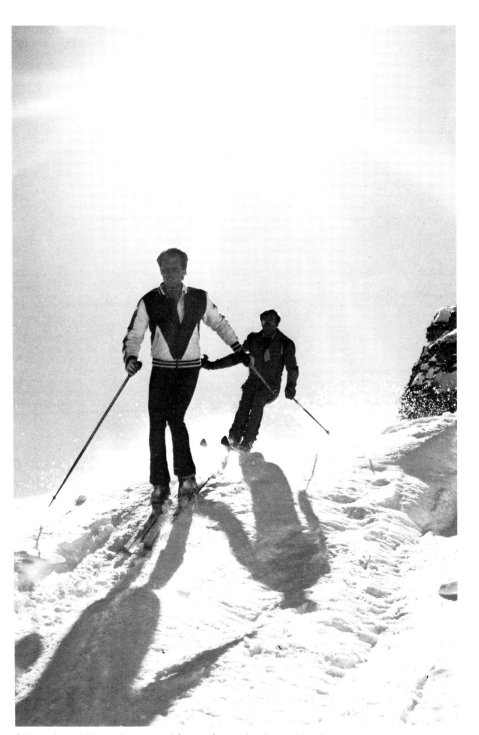

Skiing downhill can be a good form of exercise for asthmatics.

with the body's defence against infection. If someone who is poorly nourished gets a cold it is more likely to go his chest and develop into bronchitis or pneumonia, both of which may trigger off an attack or make existing asthma worse.

Another common trigger for an asthma attack may relate to dairy products. Patients are often aware that drinking milk or eating cheese leads to an increase in mucus produced in the nose (the nasal passages fill), the throat (the patient has to clear constantly), or in the chest (in the bronchial tubes), so that the patient coughs more, brings up more phlegm and shortness of breath or a wheeze may follow.

This may also happen after the patient eats spicy food or drinks alcohol, especially beer or wine, which may have to do with the yeast component in those beverages. Many other foods, or artificial colouring or flavouring added to our food, may do this as well. The cause of the reaction is not usually a true allergy in that the patient may tolerate small amounts but not large ones. In allergy even tiny amounts may lead to disaster!

In any case, once aware of this possibility, it will be important for you to watch what you eat and try to relate your various foods to your symptoms. Thus, you can be your own detective and help relieve some of the problems yourself.

It makes good sense for people suffering from hay fever or asthma to cut down on milk and dairy consumption and to watch for significant improvement. This is particularly true during the allergy season.

Eating regularly is not the same as eating properly and it is only the right foods which are nutritious and help maintain good health. Lots of sugars and starches (bread and pasta, pastry and so on) lead to being overweight which, as I have just said, is not good for the asthmatic.

Eating a balanced diet means getting plenty of proteins. Fish, meat and poultry are good sources, as are wheat, rice, pulses, beans and nuts. If you are allergic to any foods, you will need to take extra care over your diet to make sure you are getting the proteins you need while avoiding the foods to which you are allergic. The bulk of our energy comes from carbohydrates (found mainly in cereals, vegetables and fruit). These also contain cellulose or fibre, which is most useful in providing roughage. However you should not take an excess of carbohydrate as this will make you put on weight. Ideally proteins and carbohydrates should make up the largest part of your diet. The other important elements are fats, which produce energy and perform a lot of other roles in maintaining your health. Butter, vegetable and animal oils will all provide these important fatty acids although you should eat these in moderation. The only other things you need are vitamins and minerals.

If you are eating a well balanced diet with enough protein, fats and fresh fruit and vegetables, you should be getting all the vitamins and minerals you need and supplements should only be necessary for young, growing children and pregnant women.

Can asthma be affected by pregnancy?

A special word must be said about asthma and pregnancy. There is no reason why a woman with asthma should not become pregnant and have a perfectly normal baby. In various studies the same findings emerged – one third of pregnant women found that their asthma got better, one third felt that their asthma got somewhat worse and the other third found no change at all.

By taking good care of themselves and with good medical care, women with asthma have had no more trouble during labour than non-asthmatic women. And there has been no particular problem with their babies.

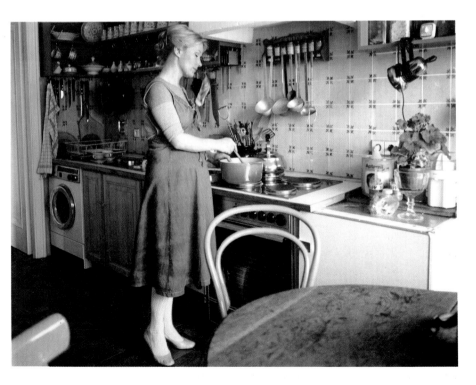

Pregnancy should not hold any special fears for an asthmatic woman.

Asthma and your heart

Understandably many patients who suffer from asthma are concerned that the attacks may damage their hearts. Quite commonly during a bout of wheezing they may feel pain in their chests which they attribute to heart strain. They are also aware of a very fast and sometimes slightly irregular heartbeat. They wonder if this is a heart attack.

Generally speaking, I am happy to reassure them that no harm is being done to their hearts. They are not having a heart attack, which is a term that should only be applied to the damage done to heart muscle as a result of hardening of the arteries. Heart disease is a quite separate problem from asthma. Heart disease tends to occur with increasing frequency in middle age and afterwards. It is related to factors such as heredity, high blood pressure and diet but never directly to asthma.

Nevertheless an attack of asthma can put some strain on your heart. The muscles of your chest, abdominal wall and diaphragm all have to work harder, which demands more oxygen. At the same time less oxygen is getting into your blood because the bronchial tubes are not working as efficiently as usual. To make up for this your heart has to pump more blood round your body. Your heart rate will therefore rise and your blood pressure may also go up slightly – but never to any dangerous degree. The increase in heart rate is not much greater than you get during any vigorous exercise, and once the asthmatic attack subsides it will return to normal and the heart muscle, which is a powerful organ with plenty of reserves in young people and anyone in good health, remains unchanged.

If you are an older person and do already suffer from coronary heart disease, asthma will put an added strain on your heart. But many asthmatics even in their seventies and eighties have perfectly normal hearts and they will not suffer any ill effects from having to work a bit harder during an attack of asthma.

Chest pain during an asthmatic attack

A pain in the chest is often interpreted as a heart attack – particularly after all the recent publicity on the subject. Chest pain of some sort is not unusual during an attack of asthma. You may get a feeling of tightness because the smooth muscle of the bronchial wall has indeed tightened, but this has nothing to do with your heart. Also, as I have pointed out, the muscles of your chest all have to work harder when you wheeze and it is quite common for this to produce a cramp. This is no different from an ordinary leg cramp during swimming or a foot cramp when you run. Again, the pain is not coming from your heart, even if this is working hard at the same time. If you can relax and breathe more slowly, the pain should disappear and the attack will subside with no harm done.

If the asthma attack is severe and needs medical help the pain in your chest may last longer. However, once the attack is overcome by treatment, your heart rate will slow, and everything will go back to normal.

Are high altitudes safe?

Another question which arises about asthma and the heart is whether or not it is safe to go up to high altitudes – not necessarily to live but maybe just to go mountain climbing or skiing. Anyone with asthma who is fit enough to do mountaineering is obviously already in excellent physical shape. The effort involved may cause some wheezing, but this can be dealt with quite easily by appropriate medicines.

It is only at very extreme altitudes that the thin air might cause problems for an asthmatic. In general people with asthma feel better at higher altitudes and in clear, unpolluted mountain air than they do normally.

As far as flying is concerned, there should be no special risk to the asthmatic person in today's pressurized aircraft. Indeed, here again, some people find the change in air pressure actually makes their breathing easier. If you have very severe asthma you should consult your doctor before flying, but otherwise you should not need to worry.

Going for a mountain walk holds no dangers as far as reduced oxygen levels are concerned.

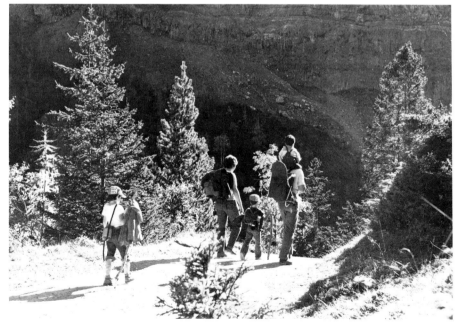

Can asthmatic drugs affect your heart?

Many of the drugs that have been used to treat asthma have a direct action on the heart. There used to be some more powerful kinds of inhaler which, if used to excess, could give you a rapid or irregular heartbeat. However these kinds are no longer used and you can rest assured that the modern ones have little or no effect on your heart.

Is asthma related to other lung problems?

It is important when we talk of asthma to make sure we are not confusing it with the quite separate and more serious problems of chronic bronchitis and emphysema. There has been considerable confusion about these terms because they are loosely used and often interchanged by both doctor and patient. Furthermore the terms chronic or asthmatic bronchitis are used commonly in Britain for all patients with wheezing, coughing and shortness of breath, while in North America, at least in the recent past, most patients with these symptoms were described as having asthma.

It is particularly necessary to separate these conditions in our minds because their causes and also their long-term outlooks are actually quite different. The patient who has asthma usually does very well, need not be an invalid and lives a normal lifespan. The patient with chronic bronchitis often gets chest infections and if his bronchitis is severe it can interfere badly with his daily life. The patient with emphysema, who almost always gets it after years of bronchitis, does poorly. Very little can be done about it once it develops. The patient is an invalid to some degree and generally dies younger than average. However, the asthmatic who has never smoked is very unlikely to get emphysema.

The two terms bronchitis and emphysema need defining if we are to understand what is going on and why they are not the same kind of lung problem as asthma. I hope that this will reassure anyone with asthma who is worried that he might develop emphysema, which he has probably heard about and knows is a serious condition.

Chronic bronchitis

This is seen mainly among heavy cigarette smokers. The more you smoke and the longer you have smoked, the greater is the likelihood that you will develop chronic bronchitis. It arises from a long term inflammation of the lining of the bronchial tubes. The main symptom is a cough, which brings up a lot of sputum. The coughing is most marked in the morning, occurs thoughout the year but is often worse during the winter months. There may be some wheezing because the lower airway is partially blocked by mucus. This causes a musical sound in the chest as air moves in and out of the tubes. Patients with chronic bronchitis are particularly prone to chest infections such as acute bronchitis or pneumonia.

Usually bronchitis does not make you short of breath at rest. However, as it continues over a number of years the smaller airways get more blocked and the lung tissue gets damaged. The lung is then less efficient and the patient begins to notice that he is more breathless, particularly when he tries to exert himself – climbing stairs or going for a walk or generally rushing about.

Chronic bronchitis used to be found only among men but as more women have taken to smoking cigarettes it is now, like lung cancer, being seen with greater frequency than it used to be in women.

Emphysema

There are a few rare, inherited conditions in which young people, often women who are non-smokers, develop emphysema. But apart from this tiny group, emphysema is almost always an acquired condition directly related to long-standing cigarette smoking and closely associated with chronic bronchitis.

It is thought to be caused by the persisting cough, which increases pressure in the lungs, and by the blockage of the bronchial tubes you get with chronic bronchitis from increased phlegm.

Emphysema means an over-inflated lung. It happens when the thin walls of the tiny air sacs at the farthest ends of the bronchial tree get destroyed. When this happens, many small sacs join together to form a larger one like a balloon. Once this stage is reached, there is no turning back. The ballooned lung remains like that. This means it does not work as efficiently, and as a result the patient is getting less oxygen. The condition is made even worse if the person continues to smoke. The main symptom at this stage is breathlessness at rest or on even the slightest exertion.

The next stage is even more serious. The lung is now unable to get rid of the carbon dioxide properly. An increase in carbon dioxide in the blood is poisonous and causes changes in the brain as well as in other tissues. The person may become drowsy or irritable and complain of severe headaches. As the carbon dioxide rises, he may go into a coma, and, unless he can be put on an artificial breathing machine, could even die.

I have deliberately painted this gloomy picture because emphysema is a self-induced, avoidable disease. If you don't smoke, you don't get it. The less you smoke, or the shorter the period during which you smoked the better off you are. Chronic bronchitis and emphysema are directly related to the overall duration of a person's smoking life and the number of

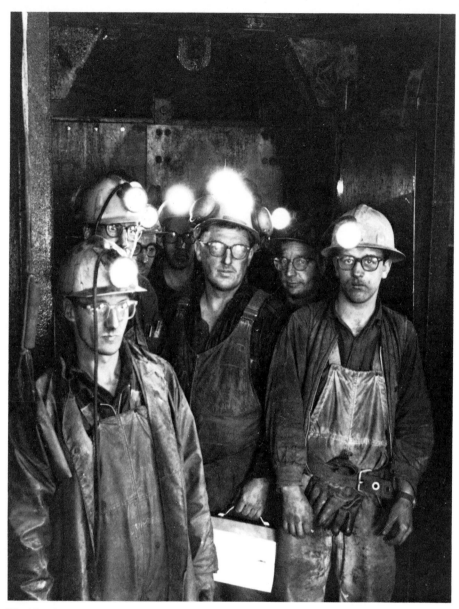

Working in mines or anywhere amid dust and fumes may slightly increase your risk of lung disease – but smoking cigarettes is a very much greater danger.

cigarettes smoked during that period. Another important point is that it has been shown by breathing tests that problems related to smoking will not go on deteriorating if the patient gives up cigarettes. The disease may not get any better, but at least it won't get worse.

To be fair, not all smokers develop this condition, certainly not to this degree, and there are some factors other than smoking which can affect it. Miners or other people who have to work amid dirt and dust are more likely to get lung disease than people who work in a clean environment. Air pollution is another major hazard. The more irritants we breathe in from the air the more likely it is that our lungs will suffer. Firemen and others who work surrounded by a lot of gas and fumes are also at greater risk. Country air is better than city air, although even here the dust in the barn may be a hazard.

In conclusion, I hope I have made it clear that chronic bronchitis and emphysema are not closely connected with asthma. It is only smoking and, to a lesser extent, other pollutants that can lead directly to these unpleasant diseases.

4. ASTHMA-HOW TO COPE

Having explained what asthma is and the various factors that may or may not affect it I shall now go on to the more practical matter of how, if you suffer from asthma, you can best get to grips with the problem so that it will interfere as little as possible with your everyday life.

A large part of this will be a question of taking the right general approach to your condition. But there are also at our disposal some more specific weapons for tackling asthma in the form of the drugs your doctor may prescribe you, and I shall discuss these briefly first before going on to give some advice on more general ways in which you can overcome asthmatic problems.

Asthmatic medicines – what they are and how to use them

Almost everyone with asthma will at some time find relief from one or another kind of medicine. There are many different drugs available, some to prevent and some to treat attacks. This section will describe, in broad terms, the treatments I usually recommend. The drugs are not addictive so you need not worry about letting children use them. If they grow out of their asthma they will not have any problems in giving up the medicines. Any sorts of drugs should only be taken in exact accordance with your doctor's instructions.

Preventing attacks

Medicines are available to help prevent attacks of asthma. Some, such as Zaditen, are taken as tablets to be swallowed. Others are taken by inhalation, such as Intal or the topical corticosteroids such as beclomethasone or budesonide. Intal, or the inhaled form of a bronchial dilator such as Ventolin, are usually very helpful in preventing asthma attacks brought on by exercise. Once the wheezing starts, Intal is not effective, but Ventolin certainly is.

Intal is a powder which must be inhaled into the lungs. It is ineffective if you swallow it. It comes in a small plastic capsule which you put into a special 'spinhaler' (see illustration) which drives the powder down into your chest as you breathe in deeply. It is now available as a direct puffer to be breathed in through your mouth.

It is best to inhale the powder four times a day to get the greatest benefit from it. Its only side effect is that it may make you cough. Always remember that it is a preventive medicine. You should take it regularly and never alter the dosage except on your doctor's instructions.

A new drug marketed as Zaditen has now become available in Britain, Ireland and other parts of Europe, and shows promise in acting similarly to Intal. It helps prevent attacks of asthma and reduces the need for other asthma medicines. It has the major advantage of being either in the form of a tablet or a syrup for children which can be easily swallowed. Zaditen should be taken on a regular daily basis to prevent attacks. It may take a few weeks before it has its full effect.

Treating an attack

Intal, Zaditen and anti-histamines are usually of no help once an attack has begun. At this stage we have two types of drug which are very helpful. They both act to open up the bronchial tubes and are known therefore as bronchodilators.

The first type (which acts rather like adrenalin) may be taken as an

Using an Intal Spinhaler: Put your head back and breathe in deeply. Hold your breath for a moment before removing the Spinhaler and breathing out. Take as many more puffs as you need to use up the powder.

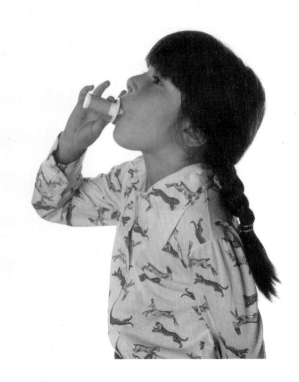

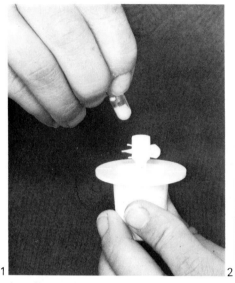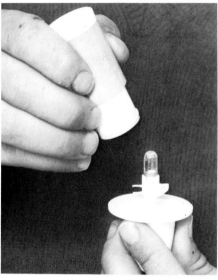

Loading a Spinhaler: 1. Hold the Spinhaler upright and press the capsule of powder into the propeller. 2. Screw on the top. Then push the sliding plastic collar down and up once to puncture the capsule before you take a puff (see picture on previous page).

inhaled aerosol spray or as a tablet. For older children and adults I prefer the spray form because it acts more quickly. Young children may find the pills are easier. In mild attacks one or two puffs on an inhaler may be enough, but if the attack is heavy or if you tend to wheeze most of the time, then you may need to take the spray as often as four times. The maximum you should ever take is, two puffs at a time, six times a day. More than this will not help and could be dangerous. The drug does tend to get less effective with time if you take it frequently. Bronchodilators can also be used for prevention. For example, if you take a puff before starting a strenuous activity this can often stop an attack of exercise asthma.

Some patients, especially the very young and old, have difficulty co-ordinating the metered dose aerosol bronchodilators. For them, there are a variety of plastic units which hook on to the metered dose aerosol, and which act as a storage chamber, where the medicine which is to be inhaled from the apparatus rests until the patient breathes it all in, in his own time. This makes taking the medicine much easier. These chambers are called spacers.

If you are regularly taking the maximum dose and it still isn't keeping you comfortable, the second type of bronchodilator (known as Theophylline) could be added to the programme. It can be taken by mouth or as a suppository. These Theophylline drugs work well in conjunction with the first type I have just mentioned, but they do both have the side-effect that they tend to speed up your heart rate and may make you feel a bit shaky. Slow release amenophylline tablets are also available in some countries (including Britain) and have an almost identical effect.

Most asthmatics never need to take any stronger medicines than these two drugs.

More powerful treatments

If you have tried all the above treatments and are still having difficulty breathing, but not bad enough to be kept in hospital, your doctor may turn to the most potent drug we have, which is a type of cortisone. These drugs are very effective in overcoming the inflammation in the air tubes which is the cause of the attack. For the greatest benefit they should be given in moderately large quantities to begin with and then the dose should be gradually reduced over a period of one to two weeks. This is usually enough to overcome the attack, but in some more severe cases it may be necessary to carry on with it for longer.

If this is the case your doctor will probably suggest you use the newer, inhaled type of cortisone, which is almost as effective as the tablet, and has the significant advantage that it does not cause the same serious side effects. The side effects of cortisone tablets when they are used over long periods include weight gain, puffy feet and ankles, an increase in blood pressure and possibly other more serious problems.

Some doctors will prescribe cortisone-like tablets so that, in the event of a really severe attack, you can have these at hand to relieve the worst of your asthma. Your doctor will advise you on the best dose. When you get

Using a bronchodilator:
It is important to take a deep breath in at the same time as you press down the top of the aerosol. This helps get the spray of medicine down into your lungs where it is needed.

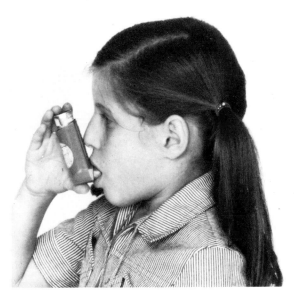

an attack that is this severe you should always arrange to see a doctor as soon as possible, but taking a cortisone-like drug could tide you over the crisis while you wait for him or her to come. These medicines can be of great value in an emergency, but they should be used sparingly and with a degree of caution, as over-use can have the unpleasant side effects decribed above.

Do sedatives help?

When teaching medical students I am adamant that they should not give sedatives as a treatment for people with asthma. This includes the tranquillizers which are so popular and so over-prescribed today. If an asthmatic person cannot sleep, I want to know why. If it is because of his asthma, then it is the breathlessness that should be treated and not the sleeplessness. If it is anxiety or depression that is causing the insomnia, then it is always better to try to deal with these root problems rather than just to sedate the patient. Sedation seems to interfere with the benefit of the other drugs usually prescribed for asthma and people who are taking sedatives tend to do worse. Warm milk or Ovaltine may be old fashioned remedies for sleeplessness, but I would recommend them rather than sedatives every time – unless of course you are allergic to milk!

How to handle an attack

You are in the middle of the housework when suddenly you begin to feel the familiar symptoms of breathlessness and wheezing and know an attack of asthma is about to strike.

The first thing to do is to sit down and try to relax. (Some guidance on relaxation and on the best positions to adopt for helping an attack is given on pages 71 to 83.) Then follow your normal treatment programme. For most people one or two puffs of a bronchodilator is all that is needed, and should take effect within a few minutes.

On rare occasions, maybe when you have a bad cold or other special reason for feeling bad, the attack may not respond this quickly, and you may need to continue the programme of medicine for longer. But never go above the recommended dosage. This will not do you any good and if the attack does not respond this means you need some other kind of treatment.

If you are still wheezing uncomfortably and find that you are getting worse rather than better you must call your doctor and if necessary take a dose of cortisone (see above). You should also call him if any extra problems arise such as a high temperature or a very serious fit of coughing that will not stop. He will be able to give you more powerful treatment, or may suggest that you go to hospital for a few days in order to cure the attack completely.

If you follow this programme you should recover quickly and markedly from any bout of wheezing, no matter how severe it seems.

Hints for coping with asthma in your everyday life

There are a number of ways in which you can arrange your daily life to minimize the problems connected with having asthma.

It is obviously not a good idea to spend time in places where a lot of dust is being stirred up. Spring cleaning and clearing out the attic, for example, are jobs you should always try to ask someone else to do for you. The same applies to cutting the lawn or shovelling snow. While jobs like these are being done you would do well to stay as far out of the way as possible.

If you are invited to a party or are spending an evening at a nightclub where the smoky atmosphere and the effort of dancing are both liable to bring on an attack, I would recommend you to take a puff of your bronchodilator before you go. If you do start to feel wheezy during the evening, get out for a break into some fresh air and wait calmly until the attack subsides before you go back to the party. This is much better than staying in the smoky room hoping the wheeze will get better and allowing it to develop into a really severe attack.

Another useful hint is to try to plan your day to make sure you won't have to rush anywhere at the last minute. The stress as well as the physical effort of having, for example, to run to catch a train are all too likely to make you wheezy. Another thing I would suggest here is that you try to avoid rush hour travel as much as possible. Wherever there are large crowds of people the atmosphere will tend to be hot and stuffy and liable to make your breathing more difficult.

If you suffer from bad asthma you will probably find it helps to do your daily tasks slowly, taking frequent pauses to get your breath back as you go along, rather than carrying on and allowing the breathlessness to build up into a major attack.

Less easy to arrange but perhaps most valuable of all is to try to make sure that the environment both at home and at your work is as clean and airy as possible.

What to do if your child has asthma

Parents usually ask me what they should do when their asthmatic child has an attack. Fortunately asthma in children is generally mild and will respond to simple measures. The first thing I point out is that in many instances it is possible to prevent it happening at all. The best way to do this is to keep him away from anything you know will cause him to start wheezing. For example if you are visiting friends who have a cat which you know might trigger off your child's asthma try to ask them beforehand to make sure the cat is kept outside during your visit – or better still arrange to meet elsewhere as the cat's fur will still be in the house.

Asthma can often be prevented by the use of Zaditen or a simple Intal inhaler (see page 60). Encouraging your child to take a regular puff several times a day will often stop him getting so many attacks. Taking medication just before vigorous exercise is also a good way of warding off an attack of asthma before it begins.

Many attacks are heralded by warning signs such as sneezing spells or a runny nose. These may be due to a cold or an allergy or to something breathed in from the air, particularly in foggy or humid weather. If you are alert to notice these symptoms and can stop them quickly the coughing and asthma may never develop. I have sometimes found that antihistamines will ward off this kind of attack, but this is not a practice commonly used by many doctors.

Once the wheezing actually starts, Intal, as I have already pointed out, is no help. The medicine to use at this stage is a bronchodilator (see page 61) which can be either inhaled if the child is old enough to co-operate or taken as a syrup or tablet. It is important to continue giving the medicine for a week or more to make sure the attack is truly over. You should make sure that it is you, and not your young child, who controls how often the inhaler is used. Relaxing exercises, particularly those to help breathing (see page 83) will sometimes help the child to breathe more slowly and efficiently and so stop the attack. In really severe cases you can, if your doctor has prescribed them, give your child cortisone-like tablets. But, as I have mentioned, you should not get into the habit of resorting to these except when really necessary, as using them over long periods can have harmful side effects. Always call the doctor if your child gets a very bad attack that does not seem to be responding to normal treatment.

Children with croup, or who wheeze because of chest colds, usually benefit from warm, moisturized air. You can buy special vaporizers to put, for example, in the child's bedroom, which he may find eases his breathing. Some children, on the other hand, feel better when the air is

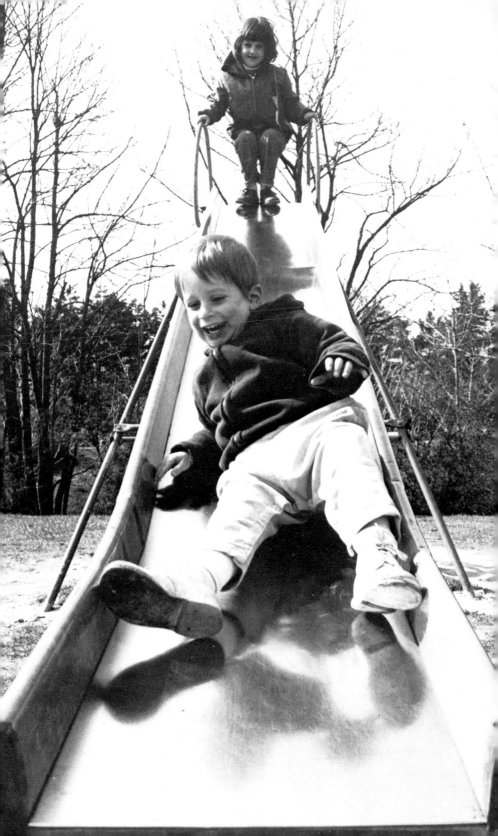

cool. You might do well to try out each alternative to see which is most effective.

It is important for the child's parents, as well as his older, more aware brothers and sisters to understand his disorder. All the family can help if they know how asthma can be controlled, by such measures as keeping the house reasonably clean, and are familiar with the many good medicines available for preventing and treating attacks.

Emotional stress at home is another thing which may bring on asthma. If, wherever possible, you can find the causes of this type of stress and try to deal with it, you could do a lot to help your asthmatic child.

We all try to manipulate others around us, so don't be surprised if your child tries to 'use' his asthma to get what he wants. Parents usually learn with experience how to recognize and handle these situations and can then, with firmness and love, persuade the child not to go on doing it.

It is also very important that you do not feel guilty and blame yourself for your child's asthma. You can do much more to help if you have accepted it and can stay calm and reassuring during his attacks.

Many parents try to over-protect their asthmatic children. This is not a good idea. It is far better to encourage the child to live a normal life – to play outdoors, to see his friends, to go to a regular school and so on. This

Brothers, sisters and friends can all help an asthmatic child and ensure that he or she is not made to feel left out.

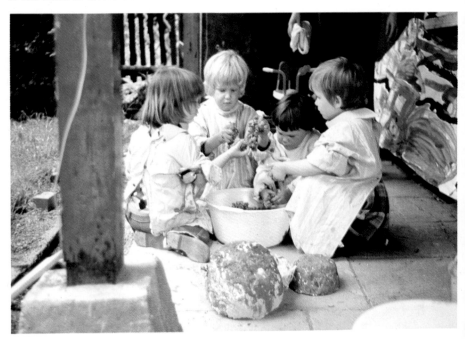

way he will not be made to feel that he is in some way different because of his asthma – even if he finds he cannot always keep up as well as he would like in things such as sports. If he joins in with everything he will not feel that he is abnormal or an invalid and so should be able to approach all the other aspects of his life with a more positive and contented outlook.

Having a sympathetic and understanding doctor to call on for help is a great advantage. He should be able to give you emotional support and explanations as well as drugs.

It is comforting to remember that 50 per cent of children with asthma lose it as they become older and another 30 per cent go on to have only an occasional and mild attack. The outlook is improving all the time as we come to understand more and more about asthma and discover better ways to treat it.

Exercises to help your breathing

If you suffer from asthma there is a lot you can do to help yourself. If you can learn to control the rate and depth of your breathing, and to relax correctly and improve your posture, you can often stop an asthmatic attack from developing or, if it does come on, at least make it shorter and less frightening.

The benefits of learning these techniques are many. If you get fewer attacks of asthma you will reduce the risk of harming your lungs. Children will miss fewer days from school, adults from work. During long or severe attacks you will be less likely to need hospital treatment which could be especially important if you are, for example, a housewife at home looking after the children. All in all there are financial, practical and emotional advantages to learning the techniques of self-help.

I would list the main aims of this as follows:

1. General fitness, exercises and sports
2. Education – understanding your asthma
3. Relaxation
4. Breathing control
5. Improving your posture
6. Keeping your airways clear

Keeping fit

General exercise is a good thing for anyone with asthma. I am always pleased to tell asthmatic patients that many well known athletes, both professional and amateur, suffer from asthma but can still maintain peak physical performance. People who have asthma usually do their condition more good by keeping physically fit than by resting all the time. Many young asthmatics have found that their breathing is greatly improved if they do regular exercise, and their attacks become less frequent and less severe. Several patients come to mind, including some in their sixties and seventies who find they can do karate regularly without getting their asthma. I urge them to keep it up.

Being invalided by sickness is sometimes inevitable, but should not be the case in the great majority of asthmatics. Being an invalid is often more a state of mind than of body. People who feel that they are invalids should be encouraged by their families and doctors to get up and around and do more. You may require the help of a professional physiotherapist. If you co-operate and gain confidence in yourself you may be surprised at how much you are capable of doing. This physical improvement is sure to make your life more interesting and worthwhile.

There are of course a number of people with quite severe asthma, usually of the all the year round kind, who feel they cannot exercise because they get out of breath so easily and any kind of physical activity makes them wheeze more. I maintain that a carefully graded exercise programme, taken together with medicine and the breathing exercises I shall explain shortly, will do them a lot of good in the long run. It will improve their breathing, and make them feel and sleep better.

Probably the easiest exercise for the asthmatic to handle is walking short distances on level ground. Going uphill is much harder work and makes breathing more of an effort. Walking outdoors on a very cold or windy day is not a good idea and on those days some kind of muscle exercises, such as lying on the floor or bed and using your legs as though bicycling, will help your muscle tone. Muggy or humid days are hard on asthmatics and outdoor exercise in this kind of weather is not a good idea. You will do better to stay in a cooler or air-conditioned room. Another excellent exercise for the asthmatic is swimming – preferably in heated pools.

Rigorous exercise is only bad for very severe asthmatics. Most people with asthma can handle and benefit from it very well.

Understanding your asthma

I hope that chapter one in this book will have given you the general understanding you need on how we breathe, and that chapter three will

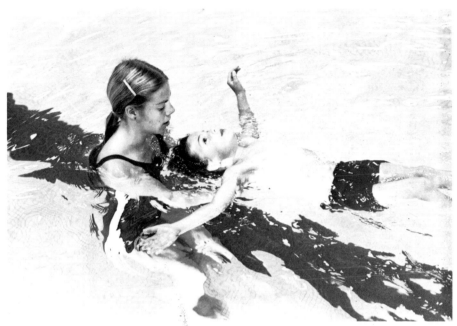

Swimming is one of the best forms of exercise for people with asthma.

have explained what happens during an attack of asthma. It may be worth re-emphasizing here that the active movement of breathing is inhaling, whereas breathing out is normally done without muscular effort. During an asthmatic attack it is breathing out that becomes particularly difficult as there is not enough force to push air out through the narrowed tubes.

Understanding something of the mechanics of breathing is certainly important for anyone with asthma. If you know what is happening in your body you are in a better position to control your attacks by knowing which muscles to use in order to improve the flow of oxygen to your lungs. Armed with this knowledge you should be able to shorten, or reduce the severity of, many of your asthmatic attacks.

Relaxation

During an asthmatic attack muscles not normally used for breathing have to come into play, particularly those in your neck and around your shoulders. There is often a natural tendency when wheezing begins to tense up these muscles, and this can only make you more uncomfortable. Learning to recognize when your muscles are tense and knowing how to relax them will be of great benefit to you during an attack. The simple exercises described here are designed to teach you this technique and help you relax your whole body.

The best position in which to do them is half-lying, with your feet up –

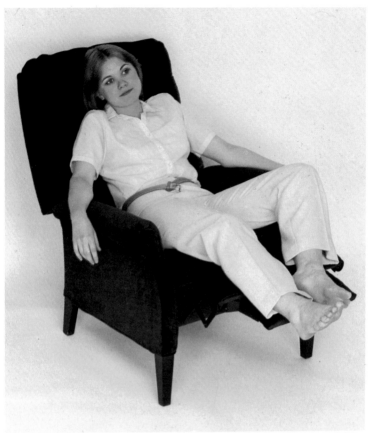

Start the exercises by sitting in a comfortable position and making yourself feel really relaxed.

as for example in a reclining chair. Your arms should be resting at your sides. You can go through the whole programme on a regular basis (say, every morning or perhaps twice a day) until you have learned how to make your whole body go floppy and relaxed at will. You should preferably do the exercises in a quiet room and make sure that all your clothing is loose before you begin. Each exercise should be held for a count of three to five seconds and repeated several times.

Legs
1. Pull your toes upwards towards the ceiling. Hold and relax.
2. Push your feet away again to tighten your leg muscles. Hold for a few seconds and then relax again.
3. Tighten your thigh muscles and push your knees down, clenching the muscles in your buttocks.
4. Tighten the muscles around your knees and squeeze your legs together. Again hold for a few seconds and then relax.

Legs exercise:
1. Feet up.

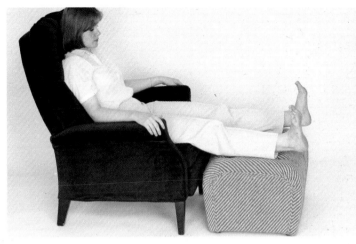

2. Feet down.

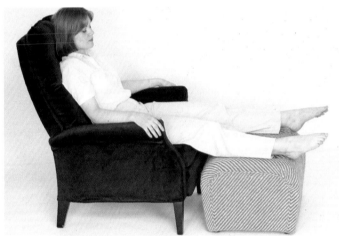

3. Legs squeezed tightly together and lifted.

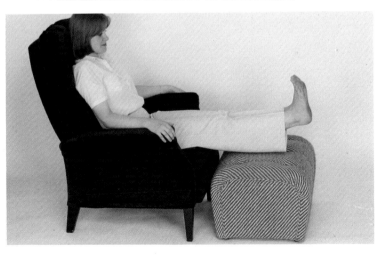

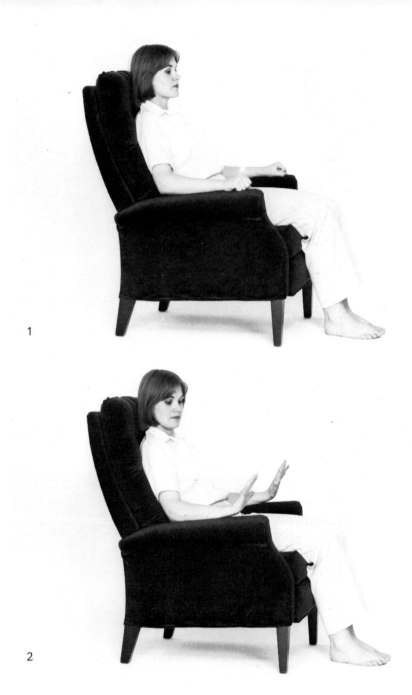

1

2

Arms

1. Clench your fists. Hold and relax.
2. Straighten the fingers of both hands and bend up the wrists. Hold and relax.

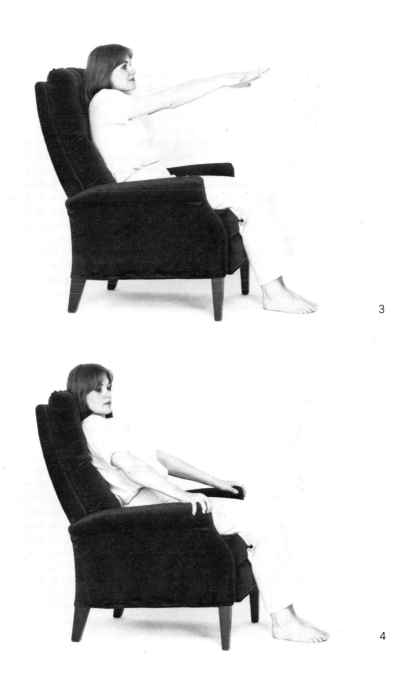

3

4

3. Raise your arms with the elbows straight and extend the wrists and fingers. Hold and relax.

4. With your elbows straight, push your arms down. Hold and relax.

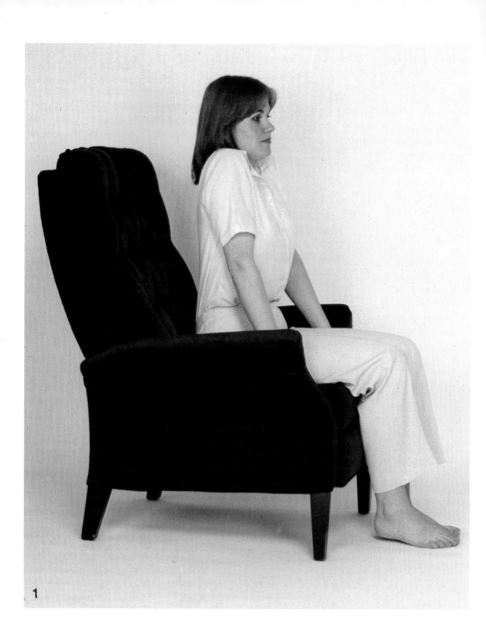

1

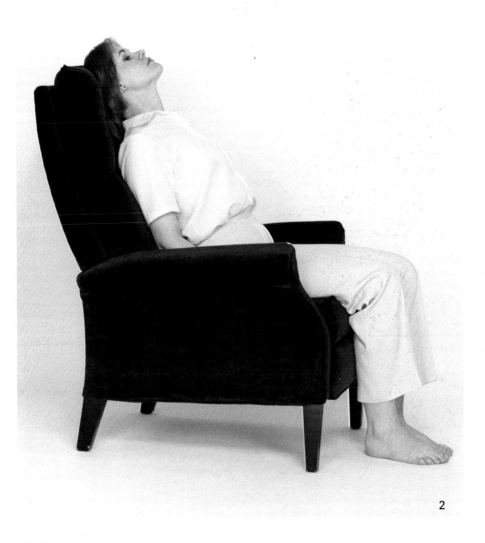

2

Head and neck

1. Shrug up. Hold and relax.
2. Push your head down. Hold and relax.

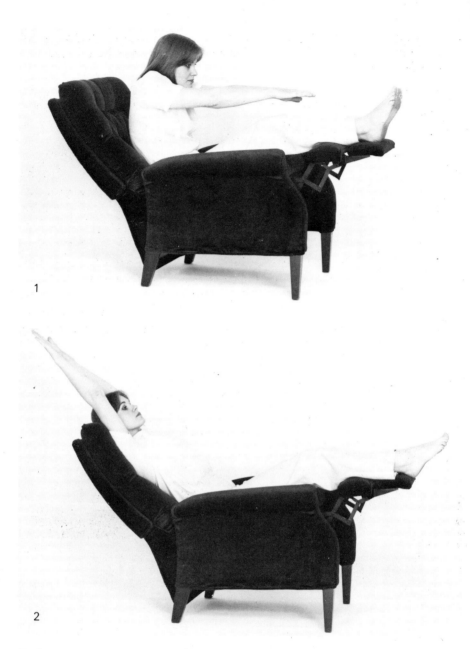

Body
1.   Lift your head and shoulders. Hold and relax.
2.   Stretch up as far as you can. Hold and relax.

Finally try tightening all the muscles you have just exercised and then get your whole body to relax at once.

After following this programme you should go on to another set of exercises aimed specifically at helping you control your breathing.

Breathing control

There is some controversy over the usefulness of breathing exercises, but they are simple to learn and many people do seem to find that they help them to breathe more slowly and easily during attacks.

You can do the breathing exercises in a number of different positions, depending on how wheezy you are feeling and on where you are when the attack begins. If the attack is mild and you are at home you can lie propped up in a semi-reclining position on a bed, with your hips and knees bent, or you can lie on your side with your head raised on pillows. If your attack is worse you may feel more comfortable sitting forward with your elbows resting on your knees, or perhaps resting your arms on a pile of pillows on top of a table. If you are out when the attack begins or somewhere where you don't feel you can lie or sit comfortably you may have to do your exercises standing up – in which case you should try either to lean on something like a window sill or to stand with your back against a wall for support.

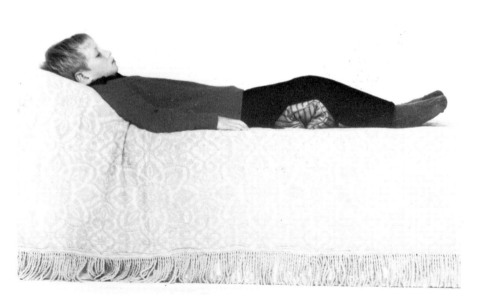

A comfortable lying position with your head supported and a pillow under your knees.

The best sitting
position during an
asthmatic attack is
this, with your
knees slightly
apart and leaning
forward on your
elbows.

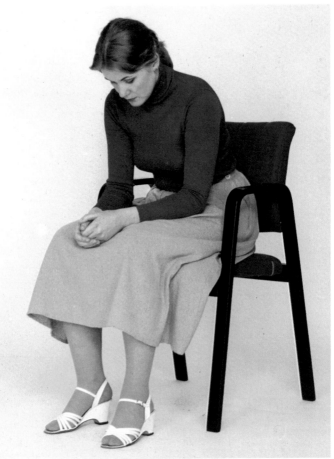

Lying on one side

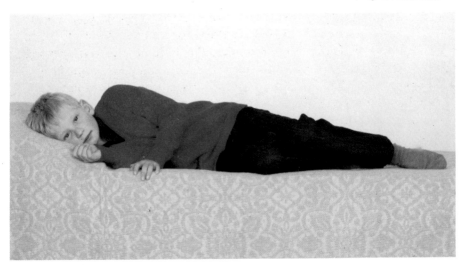

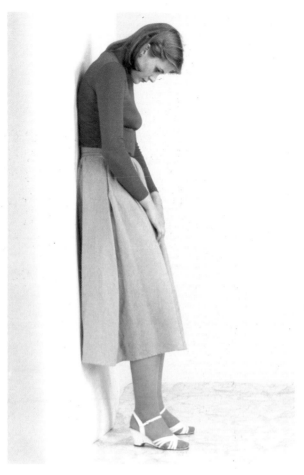

If you are unable to sit down when an attack begins, it is best to lean against a wall for support until the wheezing subsides.

Having got yourself into the most comfortable position you can, you should loosen your clothing, particularly around your waist, chest and neck, and begin on the breathing exercise described below. Remember the relaxation techniques I have just outlined, and concentrate on keeping your shoulder and neck muscles as relaxed as possible. Don't hunch yourself up, and try to keep your arms at rest rather than gripping onto any nearby support.

The basic exercise you should master is to breathe with your diaphragm. Even children can learn this technique with no difficulty. It is best to practise doing it between attacks as well as during them as that way you should find good breathing will become a habit.

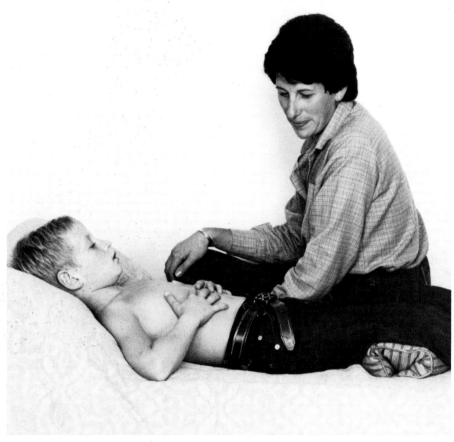

The ideal position for diaphragmatic breathing – clothes loosened and with your hands resting on your rib cage.

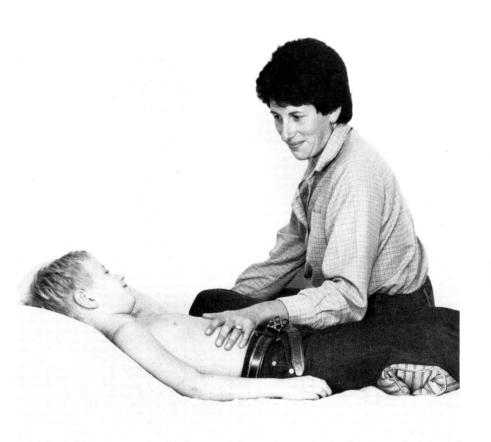

Parents can sometimes help by laying the base of their palm gently on the child's tummy to check that the diaphragm is moving correctly.

The diaphragm is one of the main muscles used in breathing. To learn to strengthen it you should ideally take up the following position. Lie partly reclining with your head and neck supported by firm pillows, and with a cushion under your knees so that they can stay slightly bent and relaxed. In this position your diaphragm should move properly as you breathe in. Make sure that you have got no tight clothing on that will restrict it and concentrate on breathing from as low down in your chest as possible. You can try putting one hand flat on your stomach, just below your rib cage. As you breathe in slowly you will feel it move out, and then down again as you exhale.

During this exercise and during attacks it is best to breathe in through your nose so that the air can be properly warmed and moistened.

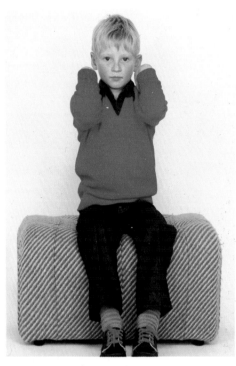

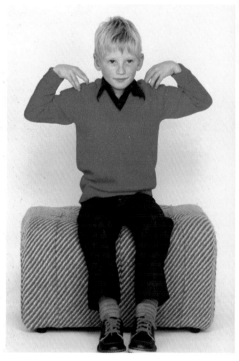

1. Elbows forward.

2. Elbows out to the sides.

Wing sitting exercise: (Repeat several times)

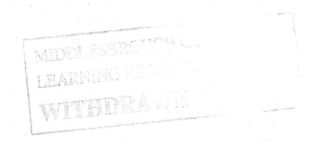

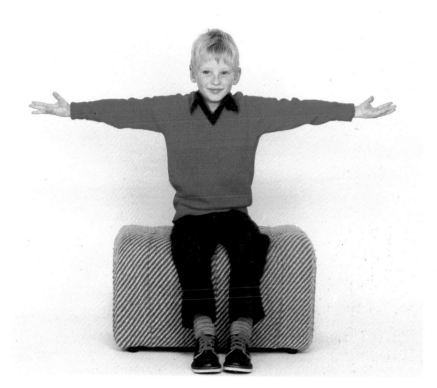

3. Arms outstretched.

Improving posture

People who have had severe asthma for a long time may develop defects in their posture. They sometimes become rather barrel chested because of the large amount of air that gets trapped in their lungs, and breathing can then become more difficult. It is best to start practising the exercises that help prevent these postural defects when you first develop asthma.

There are several chest opening exercises which help counteract the effects of asthma on your posture, and two ideas are illustrated here and on the next page. Another thing which helps is to practise deep breathing, making your lower ribs swing up and out as you inhale, and then relax as you exhale. However you should not take this to extremes as that might bring on an attack. You should also take care not to take more than five or six deep breaths in a row as going on for too long could make you feel light headed and a bit faint unless you do it very slowly. Your shoulders and upper chest should remain as still as possible throughout the exercise.

When doing this deep breathing, you should place your hands on the sides of your lower ribs so that you can feel that they are moving as they should.

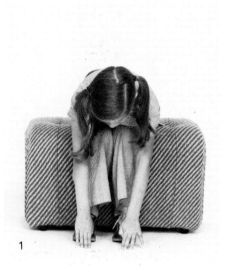

1

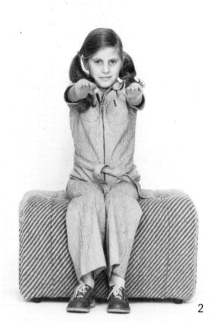

2

Another chest opening exercise:
1. Touch your toes and breathe out. 2. As you start to uncurl, begin breathing in. 3. When you are sitting up straight with your arms above your head you should have breathed in fully and be ready to start the whole exercise again.

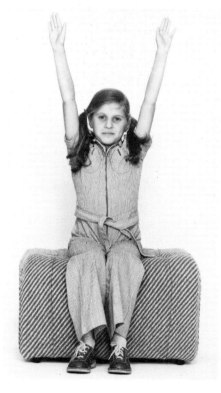

3

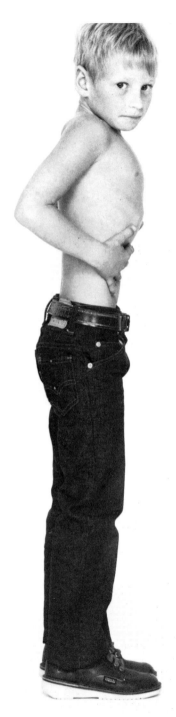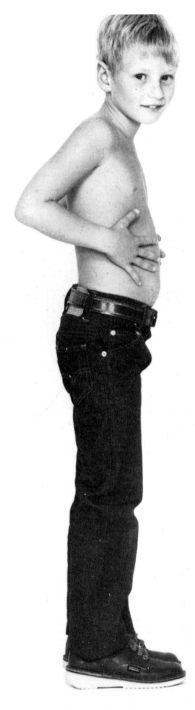

Deep breathing: As you breathe in your rib cage swings up and out.

As you breathe out the rib cage relaxes again.

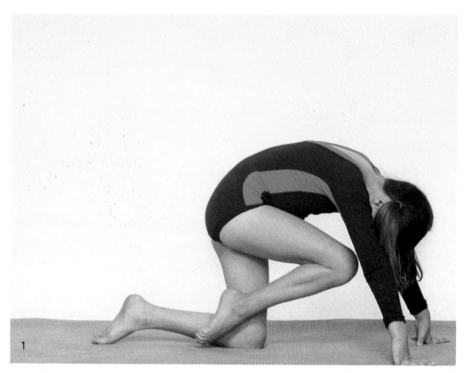

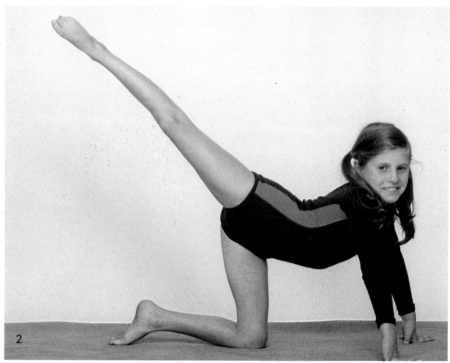

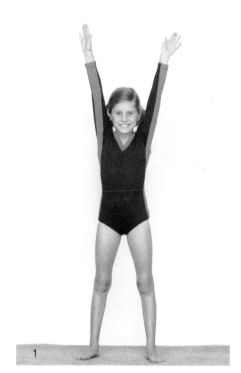
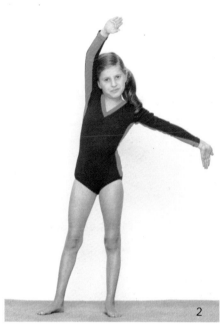
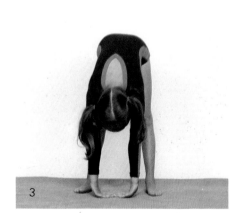
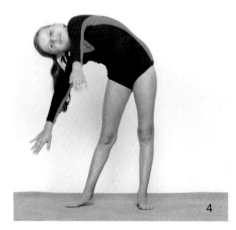

Exercise is good for asthmatics. These two gymnastic routines are excellent ones to help keep the rib cage mobile.

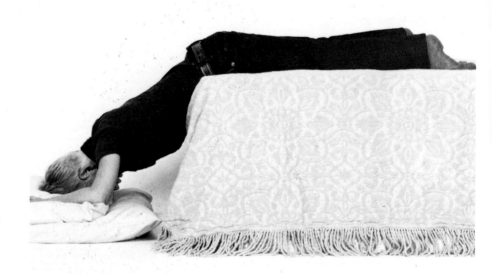

This is the most drastic method of helping you to cough your lungs clear. It can be effective for children, but stop at once if it seems to be making the asthma worse.

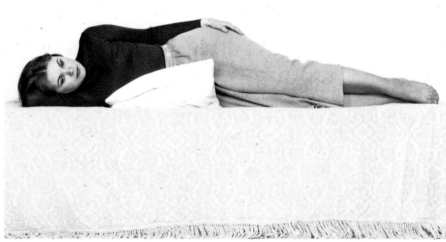

Lying with pillows under your hips is an easier method, particularly for adults.

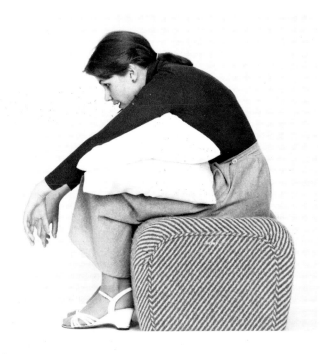

Another alternative is to lean forward over a pile of pillows – either on your lap or on a table in front of you, whichever seems easiest.

Keeping your airways clear

One of the problems of asthma particularly when it is associated with infections is that mucus tends to collect in your bronchial tubes. If you suffer from this problem and have difficulty coughing up all the mucus your physiotherapist may advise you to try what is known as postural drainage. The principle of this technique is to use gravity to drain the lower portions of your bronchial tubes. This means getting into a position where the top of your chest is tilted downwards.

There are several ways of doing this, depending on how severe your asthma is. The most effective method is to lie on a bed or table with your head and upper chest well down towards the floor, and your hips and legs raised up on pillows. This is often easier to do for children, who can be propped up over cushions or on the side of a couch, than it is for adults. In some cases it can constrict your diaphragm and make breathing more difficult. If your attack is severe, or if you find for any reason that this position makes your asthma worse, you should try one of the less extreme methods illustrated here. Any of them should make it easier for you to cough the mucus out of your lungs. It will also be helpful if you take occasional very slow, deep breaths.

One other general tip on keeping your airways clear is to make sure you blow your nose thoroughly when you get up in the morning and throughout the day if your nose feels blocked.

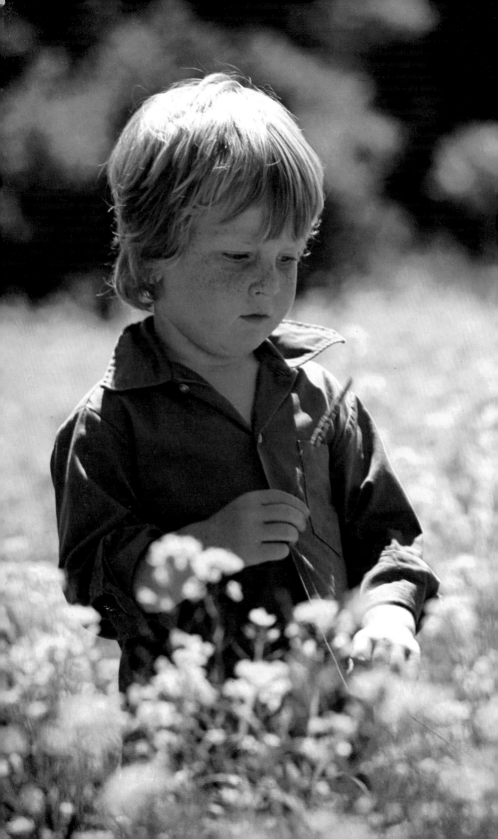

5. HAY FEVER

So far I have mainly been discussing breathing problems associated with your lungs. This chapter will now turn attention to various difficulties that can arise to do with your nose. Hay fever is perhaps the best known of these but there are other conditions which may give you a recurrently blocked or running nose without being true, allergic hay fever. Some people with these problems get little sacs of water known as nasal polyps growing inside their nostrils, and blocked sinuses are another difficulty closely associated with problems in the nose. All these are topics I shall be going into in more detail in this chapter.

What is hay fever?

This well known term is often in fact wrongly used, and tends to mean different things to patient and doctor. The condition was first recognized as long ago as the sixteenth century and then, in 1873, a man called Dr Blackley of Manchester in Britain showed that it was caused by allergy to grass pollen.

When certain people are exposed to this pollen they develop a well known set of complaints. Their noses feel stuffy, itchy and uncomfortable. Their whole heads may start to feel congested. They sneeze violently and repeatedly for minutes at a time. They notice that their noses are not only itchy but run like a tap with a thin watery discharge. Some find that their palates, ears and eyes itch as well and their eyes become puffy, bleary and red. Some of them may even cough or wheeze. Quite often they feel hot or feverish (although they don't get a true fever in the sense of a raised temperature). This is what we mean by hay fever and, if you are a sufferer, the description will probably sound all too familiar to you. Strictly speaking the term should only be used when these symptoms are the result of a specific allergy to pollen, although it is often used more loosely to describe sneezing fits in general.

The symptoms of hay fever and a common cold are sometimes very much alike. However, if your cold seems to come on year after year during the same season, particularly if it is in the summer, it is almost certainly due to an allergy. Also, the pattern of an infectious cold has several features not found in hay fever. Colds are more common in the winter and may include a sore throat or painful, swollen glands in the neck, or perhaps a fever and aching muscles, and the nasal drip becomes thick and coloured rather than watery. All these are signs of a viral cold – not of hay fever.

What causes hay fever?

The main substances to which people become allergic and which give them the symptoms of hay fever are those I have discussed in chapter two on allergies. Pollen is the main culprit in the case of genuine hay fever, but non-seasonal allergies to things such as pets or house dust can also easily lead to sneezing fits and a runny nose.

Pollen chart

This table is a rough guide to the pollinating seasons of some of the plants and trees that most commonly cause allergy. Species do of course vary from one region to another so the question of which pollens are most likely to affect you and at what time will depend largely on where you live.

SPRING

Grasses	Other	Trees
Annual meadow grass	Capeweed	Alder
Barley grass	Clover	Ash
Prairie grass	Hawthorn	Beech
Rye grass	Paterson's curse	Birch
Sweet vernal	Plantain	Blue beech
Yorkshire fog	Privet	Elm
	Wattle	Hazel
	Wheat	Horse chestnut
	Wild mustard	Common or field maple
	Wild oats	Murray pine
		Oak
		Plane
		Poplar
		Scots pine
		Sycamore
		Willow
		Yew

SUMMER

Grasses
Annual meadow grass
Bent
Brome
Canary grass
Cocksfoot or orchard grass
Couch grass
Crested dogstail
False oat
Fescue
Foxtail
Rhodes
RYE GRASS
Sweet vernal
Timothy
Veldt
Yorkshire fog

Other
Clover
Dock
Lupin
Maize
Mulberry
Nettles
PLANTAIN
Privet
Sorrel
Wild mustard

Trees
Common or field maple
Olive (northern hemisphere)
Pepper tree (especially South Australia)
Pine

LATE SUMMER

Annual meadow grass
Bent
Bermuda grass
Canary grass
Cocksfoot or orchard grass
Couch grass
False oat
Rye grass

Fat hen
Golden rod
Heather (wild)
Maize
Mugwort
Nettles
Plantain

AUTUMN AND WINTER

Annual meadow grass

Wild oats

Cedar
Hazel
Olive (southern hemisphere)
Yew

Magnified photographs of three types of pollen

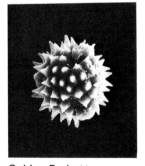

Golden Rod: this sculptured structure is typical of many pollen grains transported by insects.

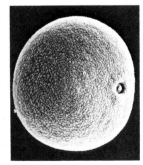

Timothy: a typical grass pollen borne by the wind.

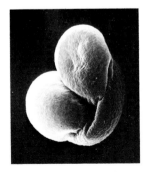

Scots Pine: typical of the pollen grains of many conifers.

What if your 'hay fever' symptoms last all year round?

Sometimes people who have all the usual problems associated with hay fever – an itchy runny nose, sneezing, and red sore eyes – turn out not in fact to have any allergies. I see this problem very often as an allergist. Many patients are sent to me with what seems to be hay fever, but their symptoms do not change even though they have travelled to see me from places where the pollens are quite different. Then, when I carry out tests on them, it turns out that they do not have real, allergic hay fever at all. The condition they suffer from is known as non-allergic rhinitis. (Rhinitis is a word used to describe any inflammation of the nose.)

A typical pattern

This problem often starts like an ordinary head cold. But then it never seems to go away. Unlike pollen allergies it usually begins in the winter months, although it can start at any time. It may follow on after you have suffered for many years from real, allergic hay fever. Then, instead of being seasonal, it suddenly becomes a problem you have to live with all the year round.

You may think at first that you have become allergic to something like your pet or dust in the house. But you soon find that even if you send your pet to a friend and reduce the dust, or even move to another city, it makes no difference. Your nose goes on dripping like a tap and you go through a whole box of paper tissues in a day. In some cases the dripping may be so severe that the drops literally run onto the floor or, at night, onto your pillow and bed clothes. This can naturally be very embarrassing and irritating.

From time to time you may find that your nose dries up and becomes totally blocked. This may be on both sides, or just one, or may be worse on one side than the other. The result is that your nose, and sometimes your whole head, feels thoroughly clogged. Everyone thinks you have a cold. But you don't get the achy tiredness or sore throat that you get when you have a cold. Just an endlessly blocked or dripping nose. Because your nose is so blocked you end up breathing through your mouth. This can dry your throat and make it feel rather sore or start a dry cough. Some of the worst periods are when you have a sneezing attack – more than five sneezes at a time and often explosive and noisy and embarrassing.

These symptoms can all appear in mild form in normal healthy people, especially when they wake up first thing in the morning. But in the case of non-allergic rhinitis the problem goes on throughout the day and even at night. You may find you wake up because your throat is so dry. Or you may wake up sneezing violently or with your nose streaming.

What causes the runny nose?

This problem is due in large part to irritation from dusts and fumes which we breathe in daily. It can even be brought on by such mild triggers as a wind blowing or changes in the weather, especially when it is humid or cloudy, and when the air pressure is low. Nobody knows exactly why. You may find that you sneeze when you breathe in a perfume or even fresh ink from your favourite newspaper. It is not that you are allergic to any of them, but that your nose is extra-sensitive and so any of these things can irritate it.

You may feel worse in air-conditioned rooms, perhaps because of the drop in temperature after coming in from the warm outdoors. Everybody is worse when exposed to tobacco smoke, but if you have non-allergic rhinitis you will suffer even more from it.

Other things which often make the condition worse are smoke from a wood fire or from frying food. You may find your nose runs more when you take a hot drink or bowl of soup, and you may get more stuffy when you drink any kind of alcohol. You are not allergic to the alcohol, but it causes you to become flushed, or in other words there is an increase in the flow of blood to your tissues. This is particularly noticeable on the skin of your face which is why you often get a warm feeling there, or sometimes in the pit of your stomach, after a drink. But it also increases the amount of blood coursing through your nose, which will make it feel more blocked or sensitive.

Do climate and temperature affect it?: People with this problem are often more uncomfortable in hot, stuffy rooms. We are not sure whether it is the heat alone which does this or whether it is such things as perfume or dust and so on. Most people will feel best when they are in cool rooms or outside in cool air. Others improve when they go to a warmer, drier climate. My feeling is that the problem is made worse by either excessively humid climates or the very dry air produced by central heating systems set at too high a temperature. Any extremes seem to be bad.

The evils of pollution: Non-allergic rhinitis seems to be more common among people living in cities than it is in the country. This is most probably due to pollution from industrial smog and exhaust fumes from cars.

Smoking: It is interesting that I have seen many patients whose symptoms became worse after they stopped smoking. Even though the smoke was a major cause of the irritation, the nicotine acted to shrink the lining of the nose and prevented some of the symptoms. I never suggest that they go back to smoking but try to deal with the problem some other way.

Diet: It is worth trying to cut down on dairy products, especially milk and cheese, as much as possible as they increase the amount of mucus produced by the body (see page 52).

Pregnancy and hormones: For no obvious reason women with this kind of stuffy nose often feel worse during pregnancy. They feel more clogged up and seem to get one cold after another. Usually they get better once the pregnancy is over. In a few instances, women taking oral contraceptives similarly find their blocked nose problems get worse. It may well be that the extra hormones produced by the body, either during pregnancy or when you are on the pill, increase the congestion in the nose, although the reason for this is not known for sure.

Can it have any long-term effects?
Non-allergic rhinitis is more than just a nuisance. It you leave it untreated it can go on to such things as a blocked ear or frequent colds and infected sinuses, or perhaps make you lose your sense of smell. This makes it very important that you recognize the problem as early as possible and start looking for and treating whatever is causing it.

Nasal polyps

People who get the blocked or runny noses and sneezing fits associated with year-round rhinitis are often told that they have nasal polyps. What are these?

A nasal polyp is a round, smooth, soft, pale grey or glistening structure, usually attached to the inside of the nose or sinuses by a narrow stalk. It will generally arise from within the sinuses and then project into the nose and cause a blockage.

When cut into sections polyps look like water-filled sacs which indeed is what they are. Removing them by surgery is not an effective cure because the cause behind them remains unchanged and so they tend to come back again.

Nose linings which are permanently inflamed tend to get swollen and boggy. The swelling is due to excessive water leaked out from the blood channels. This watery fluid starts off by being quite thin. With time, however, it takes up more and more protein from the mucus in the nose and sinuses. Proteins are heavier than water and, as they accumulate, they stretch the lining until it forms a heavy sac which falls forward from its own weight. Thus a polyp is formed.

Who gets them?

It was thought for a long time that polyps were due to an allergy. I disagree. It is very rare for someone with ordinary seasonal hay fever to get them unless his nose and sinuses become infected. Polyps, in my experience, are most common among people who suffer from non-allergic, year-round rhinitis of the kind I have just been describing. The polyps shrink and swell as the tissue lining in the nose sinks and swells.

Nasal polyps are not a new discovery. They were common in India centuries ago, and Hippocrates, three hundred years before Christ, described various methods for removing them. The exact incidence of nasal polyps today is not known. They can occur in children, but are more common among the middle aged and the elderly. They often start after a bad head cold with a sinus infection. They are also associated with asthma and many people get their first attack of wheezing after having had a nasal polyp removed by surgery. Why this should happen is not clear.

What can be done?

Some people have only an occasional polyp which, when removed, never

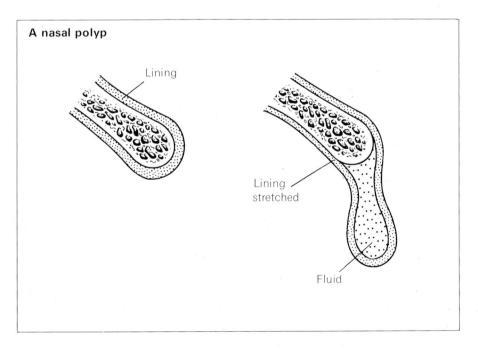

A nasal polyp

Lining

Lining stretched

Fluid

comes back. They are the lucky ones. Most people with polyps tend to have several, in both nostrils, and find that when they are cut out they simply come straight back. It is better to aim any treatment at the underlying cause of the polyps, which is often a sinus infection.

Having said this, it is not always true that surgery is pointless in treating polyps, even though they do usually come back again. Sometimes they get so large that breathing through the nose becomes quite impossible, or the sinuses get blocked off, making you liable to infection. In this case it is important that they should be cut out. After the operation a careful watch has to be kept on the patient to make sure he does not develop asthma which, as I have mentioned, is not uncommon after removal of polyps. If the patient does start wheezing it is important to start the appropriate treatment as early as possible.

For some reason which we do not clearly understand, polyps can be made worse by aspirin and by certain food additives. Avoiding these things can sometimes help control the problem.

Sinusitis

If you have a blocked nose for a long time you may be prone to trouble with your sinuses. Sinusitis itself is very often wrongly diagnosed. Too many patients and doctors blame it as a cause of headaches. In fact headaches are not a common feature of long-term sinus trouble although they may occur in the sort of brief sinus infection you sometimes get after a head cold.

The sinuses (remember – those holes in the skull designed to reduce its weight, see page 14) have a membrane lining which carries straight on from the lining of the nose. It produces the same thin layer of mucus to act as a protection and a lubricant. Whenever we catch a cold in the nose our sinuses will be involved as well to some degree. But as long as the normal drainage system is intact no major problems should occur. If the small drainage openings into the nose become blocked, however, there is trouble. Whenever any drainage system in the body is obstructed there is the risk of an infection which can then spread.

Sometimes a single sinus can become blocked or infected, or else, if the nasal tissues are very swollen, they may all do. The condition may be either acute – which means it comes on suddenly and usually for a brief time – or chronic (long lasting). The acute kind usually follows a head cold and is marked by pains in the head and stuffiness. The pain often feels as though it is coming from your teeth.

The chronic state may have no symptoms other than an increase in the amount of mucus produced. One effect of this is the common post-nasal drip, which happens when the excessive mucus drains down the back of your nose into your throat, making you cough slightly to clear it. You may of course get some discomfort even in the chronic type if your sinuses are very swollen, but headache is not common with this kind of sinusitis. The problem usually develops if you have got a permanently blocked nose. It may be one possible cause of bad breath, probably because of a mild secondary infection.

Acute sinusitis can be overcome with antibiotics and other medicines. The chronic kind is always a part of some other disorder in the nose such as the year-round rhinitis we have been discussing. When the nose problem is properly treated the sinusitis tends to clear up.

What you can do to help nose problems

If you have hay fever you are best advised to take some time away during the worst time of the year and if at all possible go to a place where there is less or no pollen. I discussed in chapter two some of the many other ways of getting rid of or avoiding the things to which you may be allergic such as dust or food or animal hair. Most people find that they are much better in well air-conditioned buildings because the pollen is filtered out. The cooler air also seems to have a good effect. But people with non-allergic rhinitis for some reason often say they feel worse in air-conditioned rooms and generally speaking they do not like the air to be too cool.

Regardless of what is causing your runny nose and sneezing you will certainly do better not to smoke. Another important thing you can do yourself is to make sure you get plenty of sleep because over-tiredness often seems to make the symptoms worse.

Regular exercise helps clear the nose and often makes you feel better. If you have an allergy to something such as a pet or dust or mites it can be very helpful to get outside for a while and go jogging or swimming or take a country walk. This can also help clear your head if you find you get stuffy after spending too much time in hot, airless rooms.

If you have a seasonal pollen hay fever you may of course find that your symptoms get worse outdoors, as this is where pollen abounds. In that case you are probably better off taking some kind of indoor exercise, perhaps in a warm swimming pool or an air-conditioned gymnasium.

What medicines can you take?

Preventive medicine
A major drug used in preventing allergic nose difficulties, and also occasionally the non-allergic ones, is called Rynacrom. This is identical to

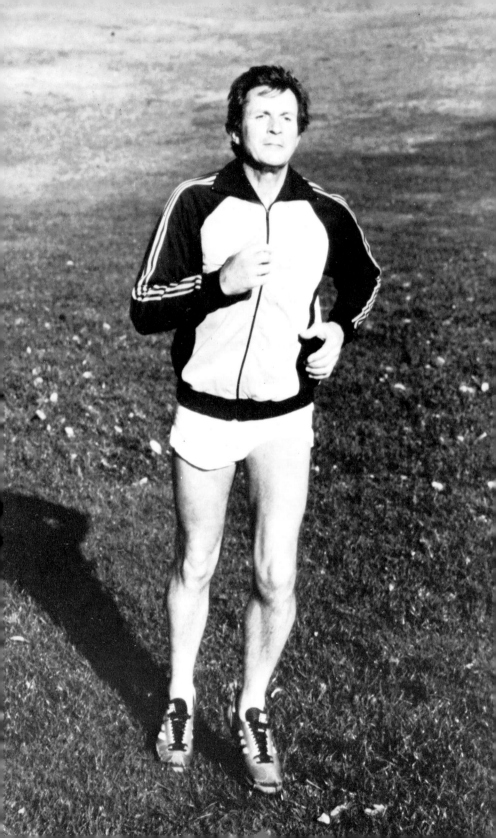

Intal, and works on the nose in the same way as Intal does on the chest. It can be inhaled into your nose in powder form or as a spray. You are usually advised to take it four times every day during the season when you suffer – which may mean taking it just in the summer or, if your hay fever is non-seasonal, all the year round.

Anti-histamines
These commonly used drugs work by blocking the effect of histamine (see page 24) which causes most of the trouble in the nose. There are many different kinds. Many people find they work better if they are put together in a tablet with a decongestant.

Some sorts you take once or twice a day, others need to be taken every four hours. You should carry them with you so that you can take them when needed if you get an unexpected attack of sneezing.

Their major side effect is that they may make you drowsy, although this does not happen to everyone. If you are taking anti-histamines you should in any case be careful not to drink alcohol as the two together could make you very sleepy. Because of the risk of drowsiness you should not drive for several hours after you have taken a tablet, or for that matter do anything which requires your close attention. Some people also find that anti-histamines make their mouths feel dry and give them a thirst. Fortunately, there is now on the market a number of new antihistamine tablets which do not cause sedation or a dry mouth. One – Hismanal – is particularly effective and has a long period of action which makes it easier to control the hay fever symptoms over the season when the allergy strikes.

Cortisone
As with asthma, the court of last appeal when someone has really bad symptoms is cortisone. When the anti-histamines and decongestants don't work, or the sleepiness they cause is literally intolerable, a short course of cortisone-like tablets can usually cure the problem. Happily these can now be given as a nasal spray which is a lot safer than the tablets and does almost as good a job, although it may take a few days to have an effect.

Unfortunately the sprays won't work well if the lining of your nose is very swollen. It is my practice to reduce the swelling first by giving people the tablets for a week or so, and then to let the spray take over for as long as it is needed. We have had no serious side effects with the new cortisone spray.

I must emphasize that these sprays act quite differently from the

Mild exercise such as jogging can sometimes clear a blocked nose.

ordinary nose sprays you can buy at the chemist which, as I shall discuss next, I do not think are a good idea.

Why decongestant nose drops and sprays are bad for you

These are still widely used in spite of the fact that they can be harmful. If you use them for brief periods only now and then when you have a cold, they do not do much damage. But if you use them as often as several times a week they can literally poison the nasal lining.

The reason they are dangerous is this. Shortly after they have been applied, the drug which they contain makes the nose lining shrink. This gives you a temporary feeling of relief from the obstruction and allows you to breathe more easily through your nose. However, the body tends soon afterwards to go into a reaction so that it not merely neutralizes the effect of the drug but actually counteracts it with excessive swelling and a more marked feeling of blockage than before.

When this unpleasant feeling of stuffiness returns you will have a natural tendency to reach once again for the nose drops. And so a vicious circle begins. Soon the medication will lose its shrinking effect and the lining will end up being constantly swollen, or else so dry as to be just as uncomfortable. In either case the protective effect of the hairs of the lining is lost, the mucus blanket dries and the inside of the nose no longer has any defence against the dirt particles or the noxious gases, viruses and bacteria which passes through it. As a result, you feel more irritation in the nose and are prone to more infection. The sneezing, blockage and discomfort become chronic.

This is a self-induced situation. It is better to put up with the short term discomfort than use this type of spray – and there are in any case more effective treatments such as the ones I have just discussed.

6. EMOTIONAL STRESS AND BREATHING PROBLEMS

Tensions of some kind are necessary for a healthy physical and emotional life. Our muscles need the stress of the pull of gravity. (It is interesting that weightlessness, such as astronauts experience in orbit, makes people's muscles waste.) Whenever we have to stay in bed for several days or weeks as a result of an illness or an operation or broken bone, even muscles like those in the bowel seem to relax more, and we get constipated.

Similarly, some tension is good for our emotional good health. Complete freedom from stress is only possible if you are in a state of total withdrawal, such as being unconscious. We need to be stimulated to stay alert, to keep our minds working. We need to think, see and hear, to feel, touch and relate to the people around us at work or at home. We are better off with a specific need to get up in the morning, to go to work or school and to tackle daily challenges.

On the other hand, too much stress can make for depression and indeed for physical ailments. An unhappy child may develop symptoms of stress such as headache or neck ache or fatigue to avoid going to school. And if any stress is prolonged and left undealt with, real illness may develop. Breathing problems of various kinds are no exception and can often be affected, or even brought on, by emotional tension.

Stress and asthma

How tension can bring on an attack

An asthmatic person with long standing anxieties or depression is likely to find it hard to sleep. The resulting tiredness together with his emotional tension lead to a tightening of the smooth muscle in his bronchial tree. The airways narrow, breathing becomes more of an effort and he may start coughing. All this leads to further blockage in the airways and more severe wheezing. He may then start to panic and lose some of his control over the muscles which normally help him to breathe when he is relaxed. If this happens the attack may get gradually worse and even end up needing some kind of medical treatment.

The important point about these kinds of attack is that they are often avoidable. If we can teach people with asthma – whatever their age – to

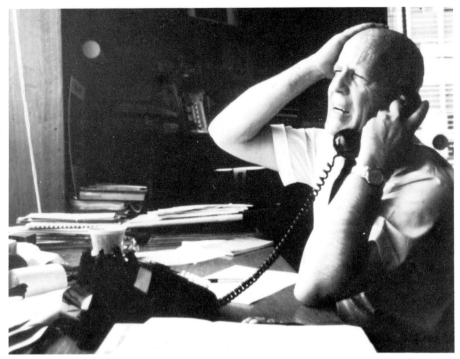

The stimulus of hard work is often valuable, but taken to extremes it will start to cause stress.

control their muscles and breathing, to sense the panic or excitement and learn to relax, the attack will subside more quickly. Prolonged stress or for that matter any acute emotional trauma certainly can bring on an attack of asthma, and learning to reduce stress as far as possible will therefore keep the wheezing better under control. If you are naturally rather a tense person you may find the relaxation exercises described on pages 72 to 78 a particularly helpful daily routine.

Is asthma psychosomatic?

As I mentioned earlier, many people who have suffered from asthma confess that they know how to bring on an attack. They are more likely to have practised this when they were children – perhaps to avoid going to school or to stop their parents going out in the evening or to avoid eating a food they disliked. We can all be tempted to try to manipulate our environment and get our own way, but this is a temptation we generally learn to recognize and try to resist as we grow older.

The less mature adult or child, however, can start an attack of asthma if he tries by a variety of means. Sometimes he can do it by forcing a cough, or by breathing very hard and quickly or irregularly, or by crying.

The power of suggestion is also well known to have an effect on asthma. A research project was done recently to study this. A group of patients with allergic asthma were told that they would be breathing in a solution containing the substance which usually brought on their attacks. Even though what they were actually given was just a simple salt solution, a good proportion of them did start to wheeze. In the second part of the test they were told that they would be breathing in a medicine to stop the wheezing. Once again they were given the same salt solution as before, but this time they got better. Many asthmatic people notice this happening in their daily lives, where just believing that the situation is one that will start an attack can actually make it happen, whether or not the cause is really there.

If your doctor has tried everything else and finally decides that the root cause of your asthma might be an emotional problem there are some cases in which help from a psychiatrist has been known to relieve wheezing where other forms of treatment have failed.

All this may suggest that asthma is a psychomatic disorder. Many patients ask me about that. They have been told by their friends or relatives that their asthma is 'all in their head', that they could control it if they wanted to and that they bring on the attack themselves.

When I was a medical student, psychosomatic disease was very much in vogue. I felt the same way. Even as a junior physician, I found myself treating patients with asthma as though they had brought on their attacks themselves to seek attention, to manipulate their families, or even just to get a doctor to see them.

Nonsense. As I have said, it is possible for a patient to bring on an attack, but the proneness to asthma must be there to begin with. Besides this, there are many causes of asthma which are anything but self-induced. One example is allergy, which is a tendency you inherit. It is also certainly not psychosomatic to begin to wheeze when you walk outdoors on a cold night. This is a very physical cause of an attack. Exercise-induced asthma is similarly quite the reverse of psychosomatic. The reason why a sprinter with asthma begins to wheeze only after the hundred-meter run and not during it is mainly because, for short distance violent effort such as this, a good sprinter holds his breath during the contest. In the course of more prolonged sporting activities asthmatic people probably will start to wheeze and need to take short rests every now and then.

Asthma certainly can be affected by other things as well as direct physical causes but, on the other hand, to say that it is 'all in the head' is definitely quite unfair and untrue.

Is your nose affected by stress?

Your emotions can also influence how stuffy your nose feels. Many people when they are under stress, or even when they are enjoying some pleasant stimulation such as sexual arousal, notice increased blockage in their noses. This is probably because the tension they are feeling increases the circulation of the blood to that area. On the other hand, sometimes stressful conditions can make a congestion in the nose suddenly disappear. For instance people whose noses have been blocked for a long time sometimes find that, after a shock or trauma, they suddenly clear. Why this happens we just don't know.

I think everyone is aware of the direct relation between stress and our bodily symptoms, and certainly any illness always feels worse when we are anxious or depressed. Tension headaches, for example, or rapid breathing, leading sometimes to faintness, both occur as a direct result of feeling

Short, intensive effort such as sprinting is something many asthmatics can manage without getting an attack.

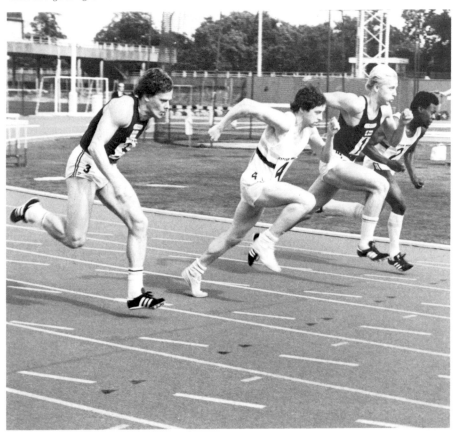

under stress. It should not therefore be surprising if you find that your asthma or blocked nose give you more trouble than usual at times when you are feeling upset or under a special strain.

Reducing stress

The reasons for emotional stress can often be deep rooted and complex and are not always easy to overcome. Sometimes discussions within the family can help clear the air, for instance when there is envy or anger between two children or between a child and parent.

If you ignore the sources of this kind of stress or if it goes on for too long it can start to make you anxious and depressed. The first people to turn to for help are family and friends, and their support throughout the period of time it takes for the emotional problem to be resolved could be enough to stop the tension and anxiety becoming serious. However if the depression continues to interfere with your life and your health, perhaps making you feel almost constantly wheezy and tired, it would probably be worth seeking professional help before the situation goes too far. With dedication and co-operation anyone suffering from depression can be helped a great deal to return to a normal life.

If we could somehow achieve a reduced level of stress in our lives, and learn better how to handle it, we could certainly do much to help the problem of asthma either for ourselves or for our relatives. While this may sound like rather an idealistic goal it would truly be the best preventive medicine of all.

The emotional effects of asthma and hay fever

Common problems

Asthma, or to a lesser extent hay fever, can sometimes present you with other problems than just physical ones. For instance if a child has asthma there may be difficulties in the family because, perhaps, his brothers and sisters resent the special attention he is given, or his parents feel secretly angry or frightened about having to cope. All sorts of special tensions can arise, which will of course be different in every individual family.

A common problem with an asthmatic child is for him to feel left out at school because he can't always take part in games or because his attacks of wheezing mark him out as different from his schoolmates. He may react by becoming excessively reserved, or perhaps angry and aggressive. All these things will put added strain on the child and on his family and friends.

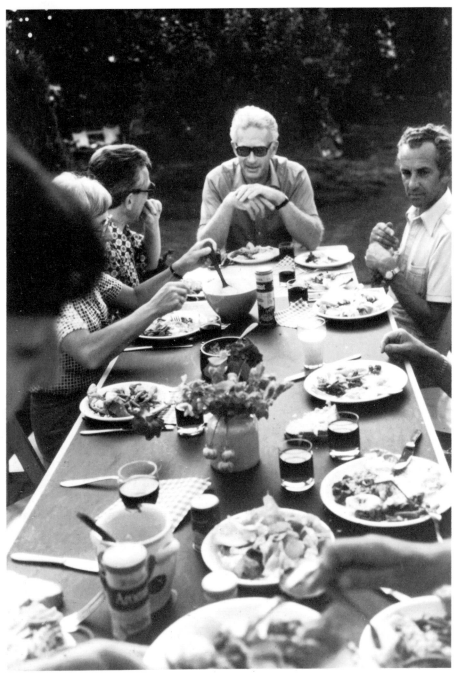

Getting an attack of asthma or hay fever in the middle of a social occasion is something people often dread. Taking preventive medicine beforehand and knowing you will be able to handle the attack calmly and effectively if it does strike are the best ways to help you relax and enjoy the party.

Asthma can be frightening, both for the person actually suffering and for people around who may not understand what is happening and who therefore feel unable to help. This too can produce extra stresses and it will certainly make it worse for someone having an asthmatic attack if either he or the people with him are in a state of panic. This is particularly true in the case of children.

Another problem is that it is naturally difficult to concentrate or to relax if you are in the midst of a long attack of hay fever or wheezing. If this happens often or for long periods it can start to make you feel depressed and frustrated and might also interfere with schoolwork or with your job. If it stops you sleeping properly this can also make you too tired to perform at your best during the day.

Breathing difficulties can also occasionally produce social problems if you find yourself being seized with attacks of violent sneezes or wheezes in embarrassing or inconvenient social situations.

Ways of coping

Having said all this it is worth pointing out that you can do a lot to counteract this kind of difficulty, particularly by the mental approach that you yourself take towards it. Asthma and hay fever are disabilities you can learn to live with so they do not interfere too much with your life on either an emotional or a practical level.

One thing that certainly helps towards living as normally as possible is to try not to treat your asthma or hay fever as the central focus of your life. One good aspect of these conditions is that usually between attacks you feel quite alright. It is best not to spend these times thinking about and dreading the next attack but to try if you can to forget about the problem. By all means do everything you can to avoid triggering off a new bout of wheezing or sneezing, but don't let this start to seem like the most important element in your life as this can only create unnecessary stress and prevent you from enjoying other things.

It is better to join in, even if it has to be in a modified way, with all the plans and activities of your family and friends rather than to think of yourself as an invalid. You should never be afraid to ask for help when you need it. But at the same time it is important not to let the condition turn into an excuse for leaning too much on other people. It is of course a good idea for example, if you are allergic to hay, to try to persuade your friends to take that picnic they were planning down to the beach rather than having it in a newly harvested field. But if you get into the habit of asking other people to treat you as a special case both they and you could begin to think that you are much more of an invalid than you really are. As always, it is a question of trying to strike exactly the right balance between not

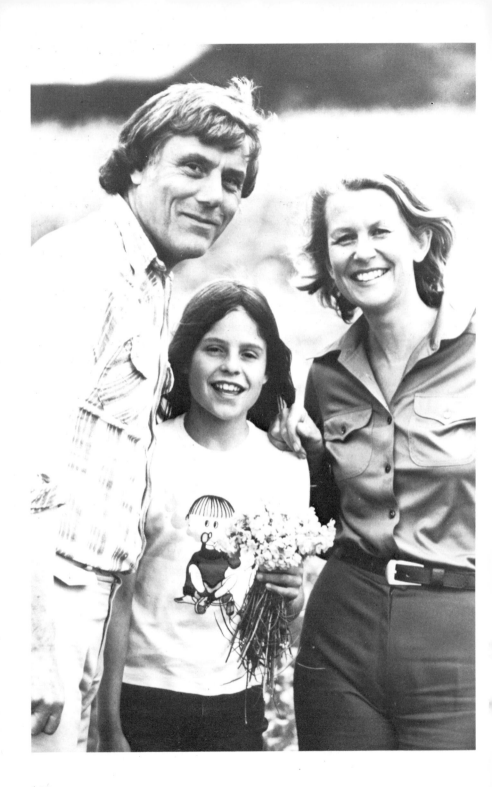

protecting yourself from the problem on the one hand or, on the other, paying too much attention to it. There is certainly nothing to be gained by resenting your asthma or feeling sorry for yourself — however understandable this reaction may be. If you can learn gradually to come to terms with it, you should find that the emotional tensions produced by the problem are greatly relieved and life will be easier and happier all round.

If you are a parent with an asthmatic child, finding the right balance between giving him the support he needs and fussing over him too much is immensely important. It is something that each family will have to gauge individually depending on the personality of the child concerned. It is a great advantage to try as early on as possible to teach his brothers and sisters not to feel frightened or jealous, but to treat the asthmatic child as normally as possible and know how to help him when he has an attack.

The other essential piece of advice on how to approach an attack is, of course, not to panic. Getting tense will make the problem harder to deal with and may in addition frighten the people around you. If you yourself learn to stay calm, not only will the atmosphere be less stressful, but also, as we have seen, you may actually help to shorten the attack or stop it becoming too severe.

The main key to staying calm is of course to feel confident. If you understand what is happening to you during an attack and know the best ways of handling it, you will be better able to stay relaxed and so to overcome it. I hope that this book has been helpful in giving you some of this important understanding and confidence in your own ability.

ACKNOWLEDGEMENTS

We would like to thank Jill Simmons, MCSP, from Guy's Hospital for her help with the exercise section, and Beecham Pharmaceuticals and the Royal Botanic Gardens at Kew for kindly providing information on pollinating seasons.

The diagrams were drawn by Cathy Slatter, BA Hons IMBI, MAA.

The studio photography was by Bill Ling and our models were Laura Calland, Nicole Lyons and Sue and Michael Usiskin. The reclining chair was kindly lent by William Whiteley Ltd of Bayswater.

Other photographs were supplied by the following:
Ed Cooper, Washington (frontispiece); Data Photo Lab, Canada (page 28 – grasses); Jacques Delacour (page 28 – pink flowers); Mick Duff (page 52); Fisons Limited (page 61); Gruner & Jahr AG & Co, Munich (pages 53 and 68); Halcyon Photographic Library (pages 31 and 45 – barbecuing); Tim Huges (page 42); Massey Ferguson (page 29); Miller Services, Toronto (pages 16, 32, 40, 48, 65, 92 and 106); NFB Photothèque, Canada (pages 10, 25, 46, 58, 67 and 71); Martin Oudejans (page 110); Private Patients Plan (page 112); Birmid Qualcast Ltd (page 45 – mowing); Phil Sheldon (page 108); Swiss National Tourist Board (pages 22, 51 and 55 – all these photographs were taken in Switzerland); Mr J. Warrack of Beecham Pharmaceuticals Research Division (the pollen grain micrographs on page 95); J. D. Wilson, Canada (page 45 – farmer).

The jacket photograph was taken by Douglas Wilson, Washington.

USEFUL ADDRESSES

BRITAIN

The Asthma Research Council
12 Pembridge Square
London W2

The Chest, Heart and Stroke Association
Tavistock House North
Tavistock Square
London WC1

The Chest, Heart and Stroke Association
65 North Castle Street
Edinburgh

The Chest, Heart and Stroke Association
28 Bedford Street
Belfast

USA

Allergy Foundation of America
19 West 44th Street
New York NY 10036

American Allergy Association
PO Box 640
Menlo Park CA 94025

American Lung Association
1740 Broadway
New York NY 10019

(The Association also has local branches)

Asthma and Allergy Foundation of America
801 Second Avenue
New York NY 10017

Hay Fever Prevention Society
Rosewall Gardens
Suite 2G
2300 Sedgwick Avenue
Bronx NY 10468

National Asthma Center
National Jewish Hospital
1999 Julian Street
Denver CO 80204

National Foundation for Asthma
PO Box 50304
Tuscon AZ 85703

National Institute of Health
Building 10, Room 1A05
9000 Rockville Pike
Bethesda
Maryland 20205

CANADA

Allergy Information Association
Room 7
25 Poynter Drive
Weston
Ontario

Asthma Information
c/o The Toronto Lung Association
Tel. (416) 226 1454

Asthma Society
Tel. (416) 481 9627

Canadian Lung Association
75 Albert Street
Suite 908
Ottawa
Ontario

Toronto Lung Association
157 Willowdale
Toronto
Ontario

(There are local Lung Associations all over Canada.)

AUSTRALIA

Asthma Association Citizens Advice Bureau (ACT)
Tel. Canberra 81 01 85

Asthma Foundation of Queensland
PO Box 122
East Brisbane
Queensland 4169

Asthma Foundation of Southern Australia
13 Hindley Street
Adelaide
Southern Australia 5000

Asthma Foundation of Tasmania
PO Box 18
Hobart
Tasmania 7001

Asthma Foundation of Victoria
2 Highfield Grove
Kew
Victoria 3101

Asthma Welfare Society
249–251 Pitt Street
Sydney
N.S.W. 2000

NEW ZEALAND

New Zealand Asthma Society
PO Box 40333
Upper Hutt
Wellington

INDEX

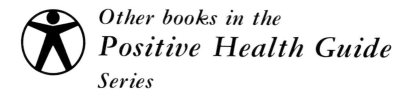

Other books in the
Positive Health Guide
Series

THE BACK – RELIEF FROM PAIN

Patterns of back pain – how to deal with and avoid them

Alan Stoddard, MRCS, LRCP, D Phys Med, DO

Hope at last for the millions who suffer back pain! An eminent osteopathic physician explains how the back works and what to do when it lets you down. With exercises, practical hints for avoiding back strain and a guide to different types of treatment, this is a clear, comprehensive book for anyone with back pain.

STRESS AND RELAXATION

Self-help ways to cope with stress and relieve nervous tension, ulcers, insomnia, migraine and high blood pressure

Jane Madders, Dip Phys Ed, MCSP

Simple self-help methods of relaxzation for anywhere and anytime. Once you know what relaxation is, you'll feel a different person. There is no need to resort to tranquillizers if you have found your own routes to tranquillity.

DON'T FORGET FIBRE IN YOUR DIET

(American title: Eat Right – to Stay Healthy and Enjoy Life More)

To help avoid many of our commonest diseases

Denis Burkitt, MD, FRCS, FRS

For the first time, this world-renowned medical scientist presents a wide-ranging survey on the importance of fibre in preventing many typically western diseases – constipation, appendicitis, varicose veins, piles, bowel cancer and more – and suggests necessary changes to our daily diet. This is essential reading for anyone who cares about their health.

BEAT HEART DISEASE!

A cardiologist explains how to help your heart and enjoy a healthier life

Risteard Mulcahy FRCPI, FRCP, MD

A reassuring look at one of today's most serious 'epidemics' – showing how changes in lifestyle could dramatically reduce the occurrence of heart disease and stroke. It includes a wealth of practical advice on coping after a heart attack and on how to get back to enjoying a normal life.

OVERCOMING ARTHRITIS

A guide to coping with stiff or aching joints

Frank Dudley Hart, MD, FRCP

A leading rheumatologist explains everything the layman wants to know about the problem of painful joints. The book describes just what arthritis and rheumatism are, and includes a wealth of ideas on how to keep your joints as supple and pain-free as possible.